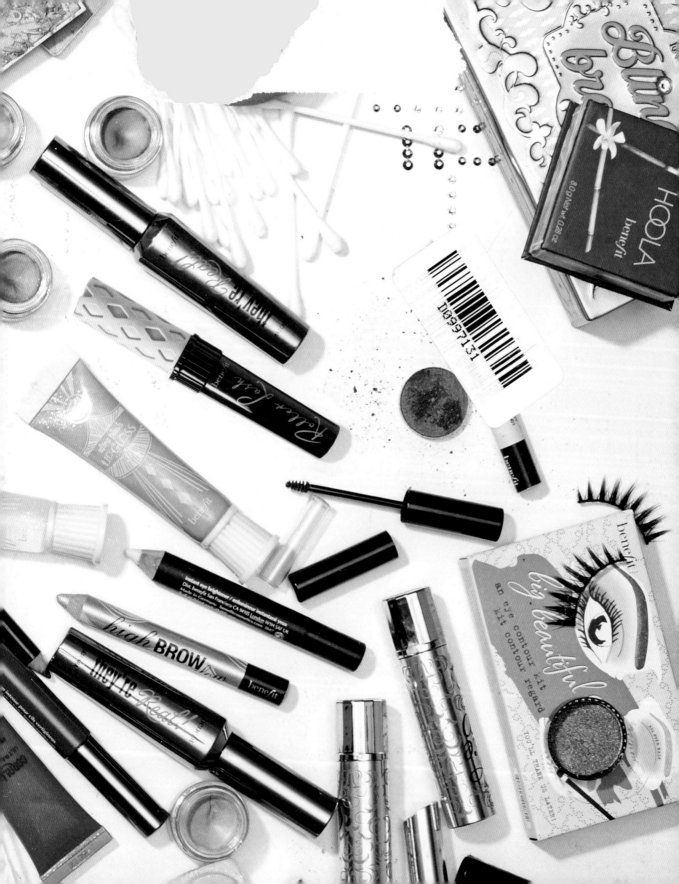

easy on the eyes

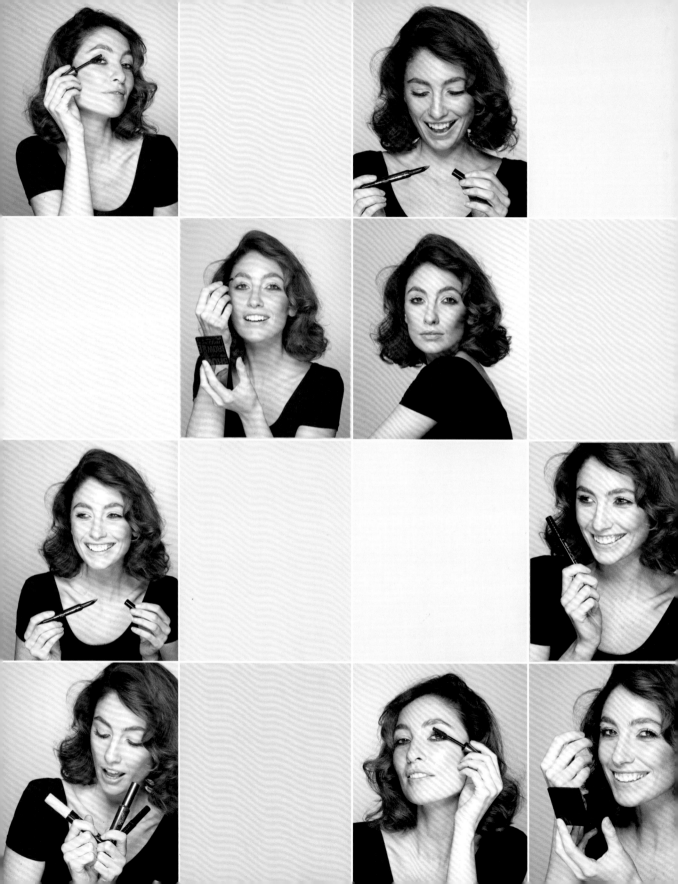

easy on the eyes

eye make-up looks in 5, 15 and 30 minutes

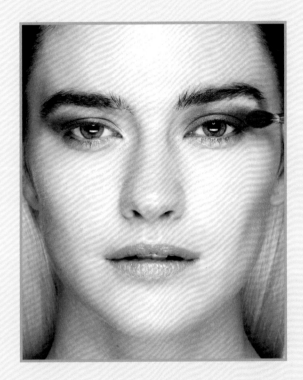

head make-up and trend artist for

benefit
SAN FRANCISCO

RYLAND PETERS & SMALL
LONDON • NEW YORK

Dedication

This is for you, Dad. How
very grateful I am that I was able
to tell you about this book on
what would be, unbeknown
to us, our last phone call. Your
contagious laugh, filled with
happiness, love, belief and pride
for your Daughter No. 1, will be
forever etched in my heart.
LYF xx

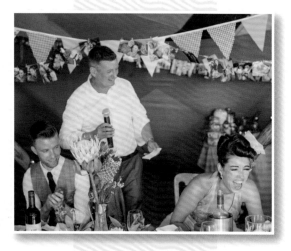

Senior Designer: Sonya Nathoo
Designer: Maria Lee-Warren
Commissioning Editor: Stephanie Milner
Production: Sarah Kulasek-Boyd
Art Director: Leslie Harrington
Editorial Director: Julia Charles
Publisher: Cindy Richards

Photographer: Tom Andrew
Photographer's Assistant: John Philip Heyes
Make-up Artist: Lisa Potter-Dixon
Make-up Artist's Assistant: Lauren Hogsden
Hair Stylist: David Wadlow
Styling: Luis Peral
Illustrator: Sally Faye Cotterill

First published in 2015
by Ryland Peters & Small,
20–21 Jockey's Fields, London WC1R 4BW
and
by Ryland Peters & Small, Inc.
341 E 116th St, New York NY 10029

www.rylandpeters.com

10 9 8 7 6 5 4 3 2

Text © Lisa Potter-Dixon 2015
Design, photographs and illustrations
© Ryland Peters & Small 2015

UK ISBN: 978–1–84975–670–9
US ISBN: 978-1-84975-700-3

A CIP record for this book is available from
the British Library.

US Library of Congress cataloging–in–
publication data has been applied for.

Printed and bound in China

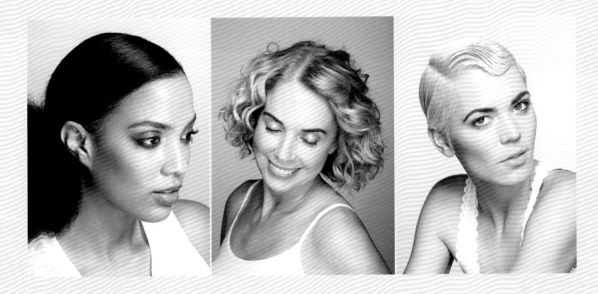

Contents

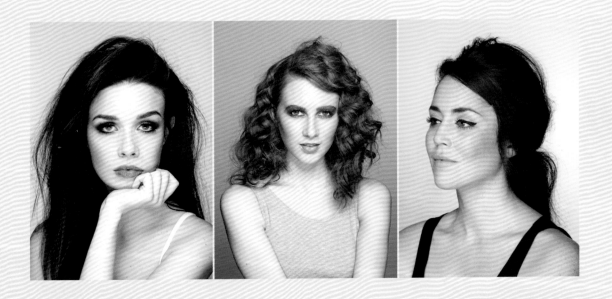

Foreword by Gail Bojarski and Ian Marshall
General Manager and Managing Director, Benefit UK

We are extremely lucky to have experienced and enjoyed the life-force that is Lisa Potter Dixon (LPD) for many years – indeed, she has become an integral member of our Benefit 'family'.

Lisa brings *so* many talents to our 'show'. She has extraordinary, intuitive make-up skills, with a natural flair for colour. When combined with her sparkle, energy and humour, it all means her clients leave looking *and* feeling great.

LPD has also brought her skills to our television screens, where her personality and talent shine. Indeed, Lisa is our 'voice of Benefit' in the UK and she epitomizes the very spirit of our brand... she is truly both 'bold and girly'.

Benefit Cosmetics

Benefit Cosmetics was founded in San Francisco in 1976. The action-packed, beauty brand offering quick-fix solutions for every gal's beauty dilemmas. Famous for high-quality iconic products with clever names, compelling packaging and innovative formulas, Benefit continues to captivate women of all ages with unique shopping experiences like the Benefit Brow Bar. With over 4,000 locations in over 45 countries, it is one of the world's biggest make-up brands.

Foreword by Lorraine Candy
Editor-in-Chief, Elle magazine

The art of applying modern make-up is a subtle skill, and one that many professionals claim to successfully achieve but in reality few do. Lisa Potter-Dixon, however, always manages to get it right. She is able to take a catwalk trend and apply it to real women on an everyday basis, making them look and feel fantastic.

This is something I have benefited from, having worked with her at *ELLE* personally and professionally over the past 10 years. She has prepared me for many red-carpet occasions, including the *ELLE* Style Awards, and she keeps our readers in the know with an endless supply of easy-to-follow make-up techniques for both the magazine and our website.

I love Lisa's passion for products and her encyclopaedic knowledge of make-up tips and tricks, which I have benefited from on many occasions. She is a big-hearted, creative woman who I'm proud to call a friend, too. I rarely meet anyone with as much boundless energy and can-do enthusiasm as Lisa, whose love of fashion almost matches her love of make-up. She has made me step out of my beauty comfort zone on many occasions and I will always thank her for it.

Meet the artist

I've loved make-up ever since I can remember. My mum was a model in the '80s so I was always surrounded by baby blue eye shadows and pale pink lipsticks! The dream! My best Christmas present ever (apart from the Sunshine Care Bear that my Mum knitted, particularly special as she couldn't knit, so the poor thing was rather holey) was my Girl's World doll's head. I swear she was the most glam doll's head in the Universe!

When my four sisters Jenna, Lucy, Kate and Emily came along, they became my very own live models. As I was the eldest, and tallest, I used to bribe them with chocolate from the top shelf if they would let me do their make-up. My brothers, Joe and Eddie, didn't quite get off scot-free either – eyelashes like Joe's were crying out for mascara!

My love of make-up continued throughout school. Acting was another passion of mine, so as well as performing in the school plays, I'd insist on doing the cast's make-up!

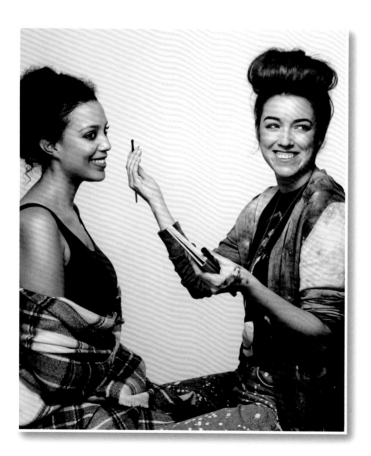

Every day I count myself lucky to work with some of the most beautiful faces in the industry, creating natural, glamourous, sexy and stunning looks on photo shoots, at fashion shows and for TV appearances.

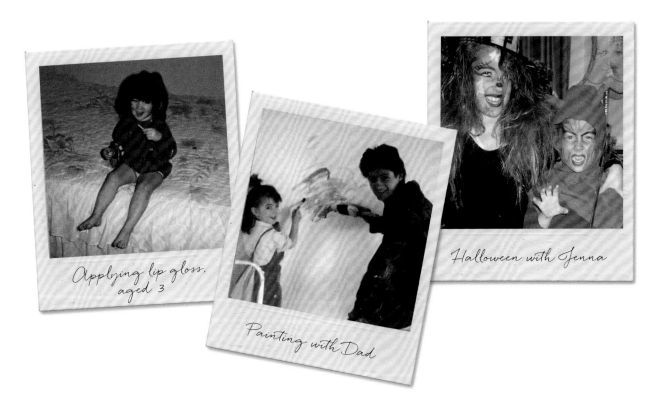

Applying lip gloss,
aged 3

Painting with Dad

Halloween with Jenna

I loved how make-up could make the character come to life. University was the era of 'Lis, can you do my make-up please?', said by many a friend ahead of our nights out.

It was when I started to work for Benefit Cosmetics that I really pursued my dream. Getting to work on different women's faces every day, enhancing their natural beauty, making them look and feel beautiful, just made me want to be a make-up artist forever. Working my way up from the shop floor to Head Make-up and Trend Artist took a lot of belief, hard work and well, blagging! I used to research who the Beauty Directors were, stand outside their offices at lunch time and ask them if they'd like me to do their make-up and brows for any up-and-coming event so I could get to know them and for them to get to know me. I soon built up a good reputation within the industry.

I'm now lucky enough to work with some of the biggest names and most beautiful faces in the industry. But for me, there's nothing better than taking a normal woman, like myself, and showing her how to create that make-up look she's always thought was impossible, no matter how little or how much time she has. And this, my friends, this is why I've created this book.

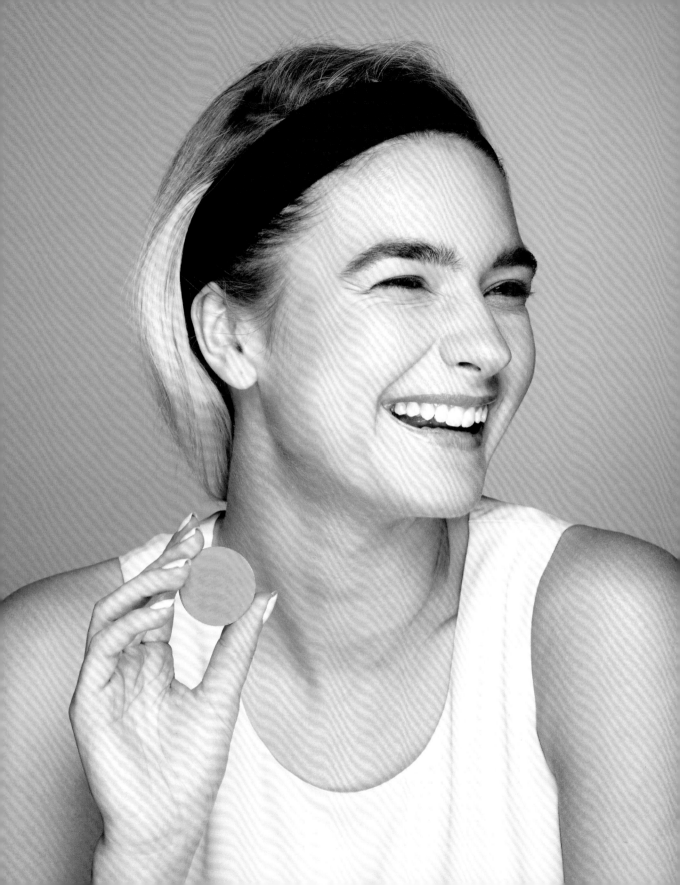

Introduction

Now then, let's get started. I could sit here and teach you how to create a fabulous 20-step smoky eye or a gorgeously detailed eye liner flick, but what if you're in a rush? What if you have 2 kids hanging off of your ankles or someone has dared to put a 9am lecture in your timetable? What if you start work at silly-o'clock or have just been asked out on a last-minute date? The last thing you want to be doing is getting out 10 eye shadows before the sun has even risen. Equally, what about if you do have some time to spare? Yes, that's right, actual time to get yourself ready for the day or evening ahead. It might only happen once in a blue moon, but it can happen! Anyway, my point is that from day to day, we have different amounts of time to get ready, so this book is designed to give you great eye looks to suit your needs, whatever they may be.

First things first, make-up is just make-up! You can jazz it up or simplify it in seconds but, most importantly, you can remove it. So don't ever be afraid of make-up – it's a beautiful thing! Think of it as the something that can enhance your natural beauty with the sweep of a brush and a lick of mascara. Sounds easy, right?! Well, it is! Or, it will be, with the help of this book.

So whatever you want to achieve, I'm going to show you how in 5, 15 or 30 minutes. Let's do this!

But, first, hold your horses, ladies! Step away from the eye shadows! Before you even think about smokin' it up or defining that line, you need to think about the rest of your beautiful face. Follow my tips and tricks in Prep, prime, perfect (pages 14–45) to create the perfect base and brows, then decide how much time you have, pick a look that you love (and one that fits to your time frame) and take your eyes from now to wow!

I'd love to hear from you gorgeous lot. Find me on Twitter and Instagram @Lisa_Benefit or add #EasyOnTheEyes to your posts.

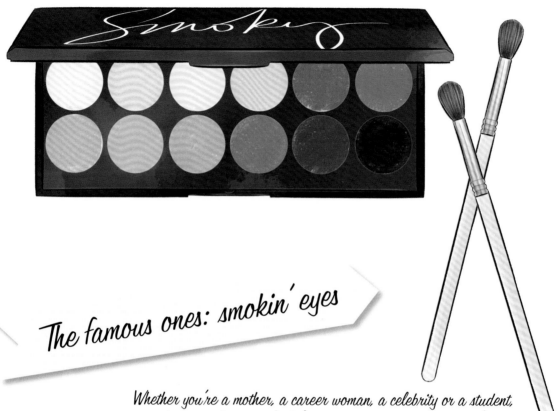

The famous ones: smokin' eyes

Whether you're a mother, a career woman, a celebrity or a student, a smoky eye is the go-to look for most women and it has been for a very, very long time!

A smoky eye is sexy and feminine, and it really does suit everyone, so it's no wonder that it's so popular with women the world over. It's hard to say how, why or when the smoky eye came about. However, we can go back some 3,000–5,000 years to the civilizations of North Africa, the Middle East, the Indus Valley and India, as what we do know is that modern archaeologists have found small containers of black powder, or *kajal*, together with thin applicator sticks used to paint the eye. Incredible!

These days, a smoky eye is a celeb favourite. I feel like it's always made out to be much more complicated than it actually is. The smoky eye is not about the colours you use or how much shadow you apply; it's all about the technique.

Skip to pages 46–87 to find out how to perfect it in no time at all.

The famous ones: liner looks

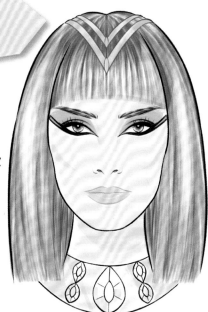

Eye liner has one of the longest historic cosmetic timelines and has framed and defined women's eyes for pretty much forever!

Worn for thousands of years, eye liner has one of the longest historic cosmetic timelines.

Eye liner was first used in Ancient Egypt and Mesopotamia as a dark black line around the eyes. As early as 10,000 BC, Egyptians wore eyeliner, not only to look good, but also to protect the wearer from the 'evil eye'. They produced liner with a variety of materials including copper ore and beetles' blood! It was when Tutankhamen's tomb was discovered in the 1920s that eyeliner was introduced to the modern world.

The '20s saw many amazing changes in women's fashion. This led to women feeling freer to apply make-up more liberally. Mostly, liner was used to frame the entire eye. In the 1950s, sexy cat eyes were made famous on the big screen. Hollywood icons, including Marilyn Monroe, Rita Hayworth and of course Audrey Hepburn, made this look the biggest make-up trend of the era. In the 1960s, a love for geometric patterns spilled over from clothes to make-up. Eyeliner was used to create thick black and white lines that framed and defined the eye. Made famous by model Twiggy, this was known as the 'London look'.

In the late twentieth and early twenty-first centuries, eye liner became commonly used as part of a daily make-up routine to define the eye or create the look of a wider or smaller eye. Although, saying that, we do tend to revisit the looks of the past. After all, trends always come back around!

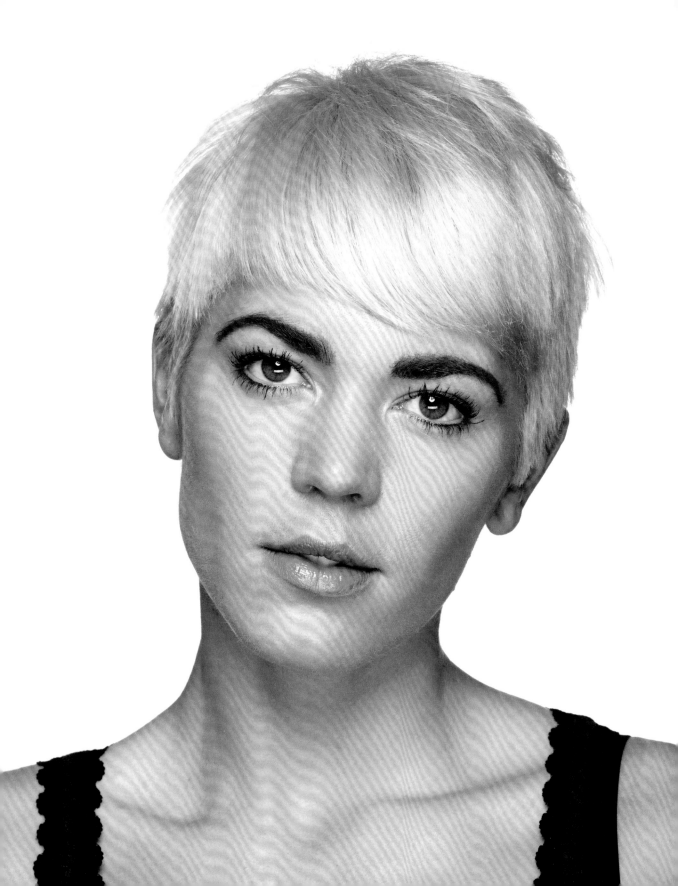

Prep, prime, perfect

Before we begin with our eye looks, it's important to get the perfect base and brows. There's no point creating a wonderful smoky eye or a classic liner flick if you have uneven-looking skin, or brows as wild as Groucho Marx's! In this section, I'll teach your how to prep, prime and perfect your skin to enhance your natural beauty. And then we'll move on to wow those brows. Okay, let's go!

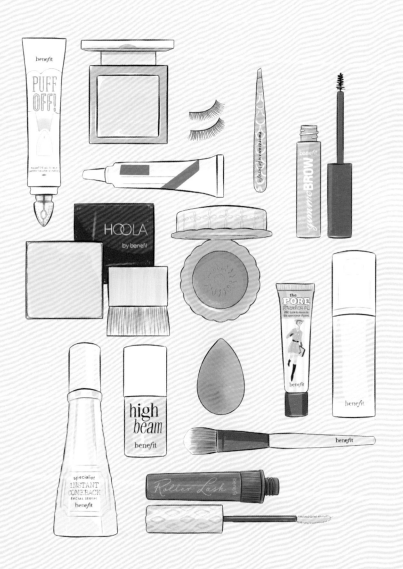

Prepping your face

When I was 14, my Nan told me that sleeping in your make-up added 8 days(!) to the age of your skin. That meant that if I slept in my make-up for 45 days, I'd look a whole year older! I've been cleansing and moisturizing morning and night ever since. Looking after your skin creates the perfect blank canvas for applying make-up, but it also keeps you looking young, fresh and hydrated. My Nan is 84 but looks 64, so I'd believe her if I were you!

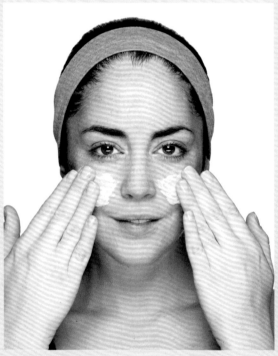
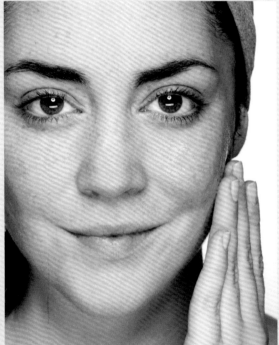

Step 1

Cleanse your skin. You should wash your face with a good cleanser first thing in the morning and last thing at night to remove any baddies that collect on the surface of the skin and to keep your skin looking radiant. Start with your cheeks and gently rub the cleanser all over the face in circular motions, then rinse off.

Step 2

If you're in your mid-twenties or older, serum should be your best friend. Applying serum is a commonly missed step, but an important one. Using a serum before moisturizing infuses additional rich vitamins and minerals into your skin. Prevention is also better than cure. Apply a thin layer all over the face using fingertips.

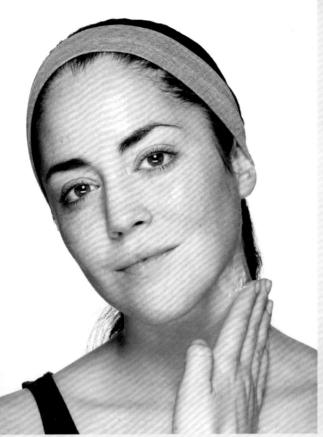
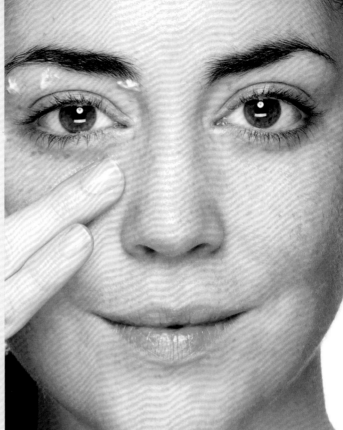

Step 3

Moisturizer is a vital step for keeping your skin hydrated. Use a moisturizer that suits your skin type. Always use one that has SPF sun protection, too, or better still, apply a separate SPF cream. Spend a good 30 seconds massaging the cream into your skin. And don't forget about your neck and your jawline.

Step 4

Our eye area is 40 per cent thinner than anywhere else on the face. I suggest using eye cream from around your mid-twenties. Gently apply it in a circle around the eye, let it sink in for a few seconds and then pat in using your ring finger, as this will give you the softest touch. You're now prepped and ready to prime!

Coconut oil

Use coconut oil as a sleep-in face mask once a week. It's jam-packed with good fats and vitamins. I smear it on my face whenever my skin is feeling dry.

Applying primer

Until a few years ago primer was a make-up artist's secret. Now, the secret is out and it's about prime! My favourite primers are silicone-based. These minimize the appearance of pores and fine lines, giving you a smooth, even base ready for foundation. If your skin is in need of a brightening boost, look for a brightening primer with reflective compounds.

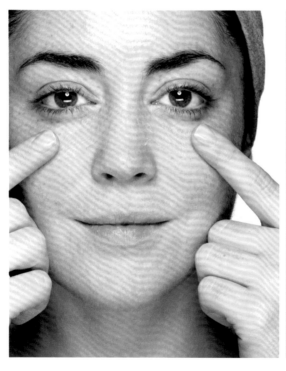

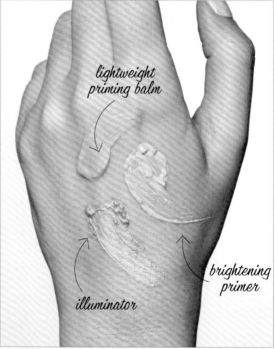

lightweight priming balm

brightening primer

illuminator

Step 1

Apply primer to the whole face using fingertips; start in the centre of your face and blend outwards. You only need a thin layer, so start with a little product and build it up. Trust me, once you start, you'll always find time to prime!

Step 2

Apply a little extra primer on areas with fine lines or open pores. Priming balms like Benefit's the POREfessional minimize the appearance of both, while reflective primers like Benefit's That Gal and Girl Meets Pearl brighten skin tones.

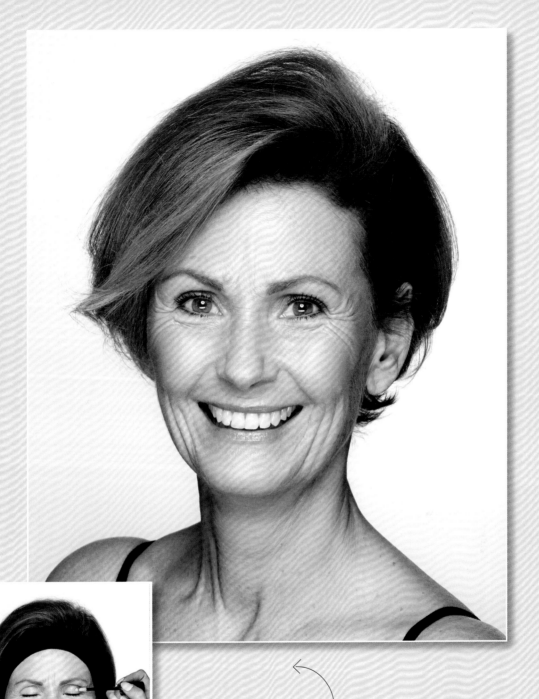

On older eyes, apply a liquid highlighting primer over the lids for wider, brighter eyes. Dot the primer all over the lids and blend with your ring finger for a soft touch.

Perfecting your base

There are hundreds of different types of base products out there. From liquid foundations to tinted moisturizers, minerals and powders, I could easily write another book on them! Instead, I'm going to teach you the essentials of how to pick and apply your perfect base.

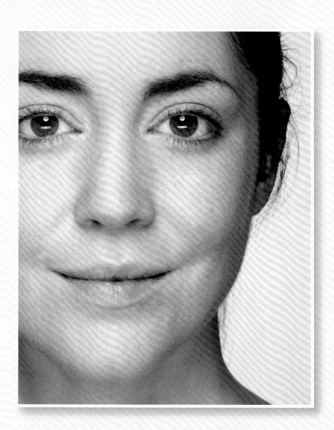

Ask the expert

Pop to your local make-up counter and get a beauty expert to colour-match your skin tone to specific products. Getting the right colour of foundation can be tough by yourself, so don't be afraid to ask for help.

Natural light

If you're able to visit a make-up counter, once the foundation is applied, pop outside into the natural light before you buy. Take a look in a mirror (or take a selfie on your phone) to double check that the colour is right for you.

Don't go heavy

The worst mistake you can make is going for a foundation that's too heavy. We all have problem areas that we want to mask, but I always suggest going for a light foundation. This way, your skin will still look dewy and radiant, and you can use concealer to target problem areas.

If in doubt...

Go for a tinted moisturizer or liquid foundation, as these tend to look more natural than pressed or mineral powders.

Applying foundation

Everyone has a preferred technique for applying foundation. Whether you use a brush, a sponge or your fingers, there's not really any right or wrong tool. Personally, I like to use a foundation brush, as I find I get a more even and long-lasting finish. Foundation brushes also tend to be made of synthetic hair, meaning that they don't soak up your product like a sponge would or your fingers do.

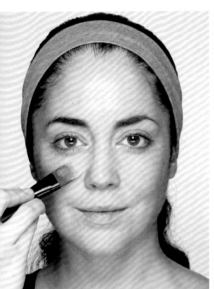 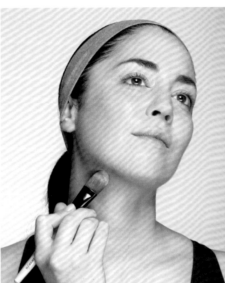 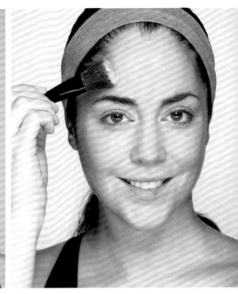

Step 1

Start by applying a small amount of foundation in the centre of your face using a foundation brush and blending outwards. Our problem areas tend to be in the inner circle of our face, so starting in the centre helps to target these things and also means that there won't be tonnes of foundation left when you reach your hairline. There's nothing worse than an obvious line around face.

Step 2

Blend the foundation down onto the neck to make sure it matches your face. If you have any problem areas you want to pinpoint with concealer, now's the time. For specific complaints (dark circles, sun spots, blemishes and more), turn to pages 22–23 to see my top tips for hiding little beasties.

Step 3

If you tend to get a bit shiny, now's the time to use a finishing powder. Don't just throw this all over your face – it's tempting, I know! Take a fluffy blending brush, dip it into your powder and lightly buff it onto the shiny areas. These tend to be in the T-zone and around the nose. And there you have it: perfect foundation to start adding colour to. Someone pass me a bronzer, a blusher and some eye shadow, quick!

Concealer

Thank goodness for concealer! A good concealer has hidden the signs of many a late night. As with foundation, there are hundreds of them out there. Don't fall into the trap of mistaking a highlighter for a concealer – trust me, it's an easy mistake to make. Highlighters won't conceal, they will only brighten the area, often making the problem more visible. Here are my personal rules for picking the right concealer for the right problem and the right one just for you.

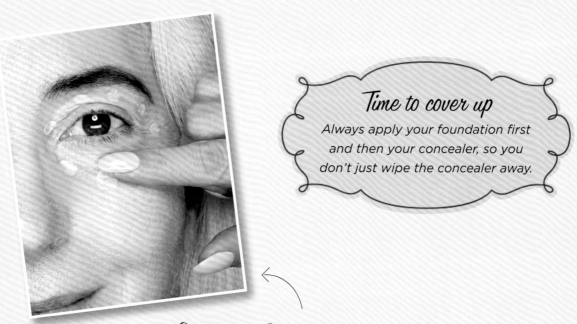

Time to cover up

Always apply your foundation first and then your concealer, so you don't just wipe the concealer away.

On older eyes, I love to mix an eye cream and a cream concealer together, for coverage that won't crease.

Dark circles

Many women are prone to dark circles. Sometimes it's genetic, sometimes it's because you're dehydrated, sometimes it's just because you're plain old tired! Choosing a concealer one shade lighter than your skin tone is the best way to cover darkness. Neutral beige to slightly yellow shades look best, regardless of where they are applied. A liquid concealer is better under the eye than a cream concealer, as it you can build it up and it won't sit or crease as much as a thicker cream concealer would in that area. Dot the concealer in a full circle around the eye. You want to conceal your eyelid too, so that the whole eye area is even and flawless. This will also prime your lids ready for eyeshadow. Blend the dots together using your index finger for precision.

Sun spots and pigmentation

As we get older, we tend to find that we get brown spots on our face, mainly caused by sun damage. This is why it is *so* important to use a SPF sun protection cream! To cover these annoying areas, you need to use a medium-coverage, creamy concealer that is the same colour as your foundation. I love to apply this with a hard-angled brush, using the tip of the brush to pinpoint the area I want to cover. Apply a small amount of concealer to the area with precision, then blend the concealer with a fluffy shadow brush for an airbrush finish. You can apply a couple of layers using this technique, if necessary.

Blemishes

Spots have been the bane of all of our lives at some point! As women, we tend to get blemishes on the bottom half of our face, mainly the chin area. What we think is the size of Mount Etna may only be the size of a pinhead, but, either way, there is nothing worse than feeling self-conscious. Cream concealers are the best way to go here. Antibacterial cream concealers are even better, as they will help to reduce the size of the blemish. Use a hard-angled brush for applying concealer here and not your fingers, as they can make things worse because your fingertips are oily. Dot a small amount of concealer around the blemish and in the centre. Blend using a clean fluffy shadow brush. Make sure you blend the edges for a flawless finish. Repeat as required.

Redness and rosacea

Redness on the face can be very frustrating. A yellow-based concealer is the best way to cover redness, but don't go crazy, as you don't want the yellow to show through. I suggest using a sponge to apply this type of concealer and it is the only concealer that I would suggest using under your base. Pat the concealer onto any red areas in thin layers. Once you have a light coverage, apply your foundation following the instructions on pages 20–21. Next, apply a cream concealer the same colour as your skin tone to set the base.

Laughter lines

Hydration is key to covering these areas. The last thing you want is a heavy concealer creasing and sitting under your eyes. Use a hydrating, liquid-based concealer that is one shade lighter than your skin tone. Draw a triangle under the eye and out, up to the corner of the brow. Blend inwards, towards your eye, using your ring finger.

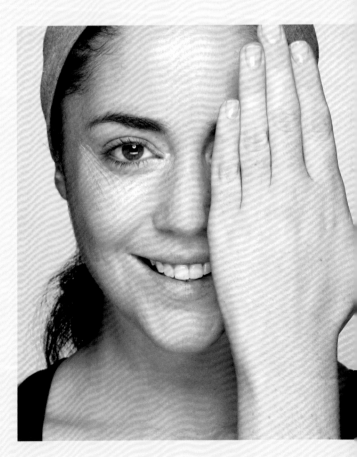

A pop of colour

Bronzer and blusher are a girl's best friend. I feel pretty much naked without a pink cheek! First, let's get something straight: you can absolutely wear both bronzer *and* blusher. In fact, you should! Bronzer first and blusher after. Here's how...

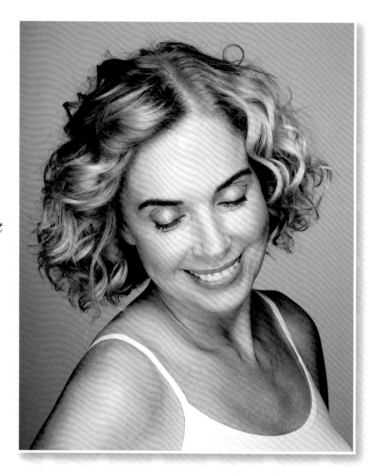

Bronzers without a shimmer will give you a more natural finish

Bronzer

We all feel better after a bit of sun. Whether it's after an exotic holiday or an hour in the back garden, a touch of colour makes us look and feel healthy (although don't forget your SPF!). Bronzer is the perfect product to give you that glow. It can also enhance the shape of your face instantly.

Using a blusher brush, apply your bronzer in a figure of '3' either side of your face. Sweep a little down the centre of your nose and repeat until you have a depth of colour you're happy with. Sweep the bronzer under your jaw bone and down the centre of your neck. This is important, as there's nothing more obvious than a bronzed face and a white neck!

Blusher

Okay, so there are three types of blusher: powders, creams and stains. I tend to switch between all three, depending on what finish I want for each specific look.

A powder blush is great because you can build it up. You also have the option of choosing a matte version or one with highlighting particles in it. Apply this with a blusher brush.

A cream blush gives you a lovely sheen, and the pigment is quite strong, so less is more here. Apply this with your fingertips.

A stain lasts on the skin all day and is buildable. They usually come with a brush applicator that you can use, then blend with your fingertips.

The best way to apply blusher is to smile, apply the blush on the apples of your cheeks (that lovely chubby bit that your Nan always used to pinch!) and then brush or blend the blusher up towards the tops of your ears using the best tool for each type of blush. By applying at this angle you will emphasize your cheekbones. And, why not? They're fabulous!

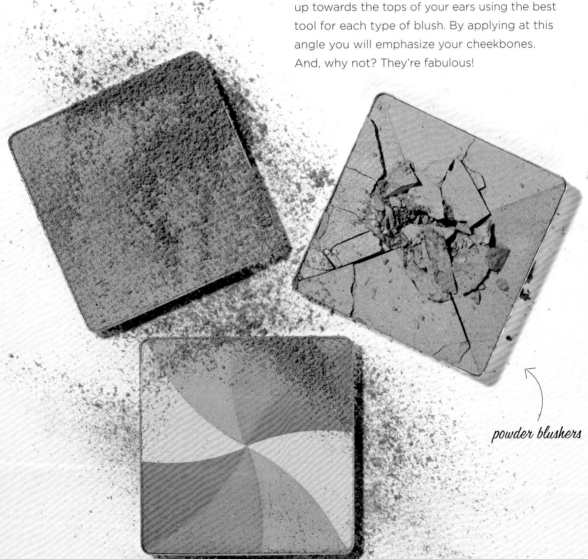

powder blushers

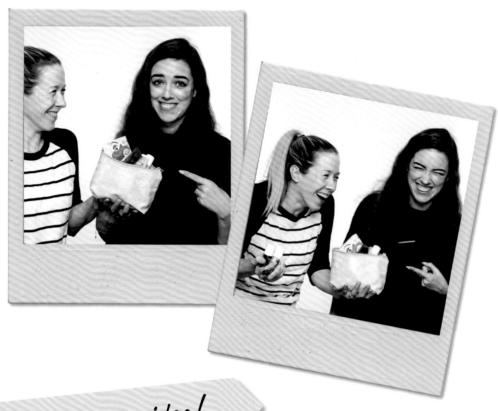

All the gear, no idea!

This is my best friend, Rosie.

We've been friends for 15 years. Now she doesn't mind me telling you this, but Rosie has worn the same three make-up products for the past 17 years! Two of these happen to be Benefit products: Benetint lip and cheek stain and High Beam highlighter. The third is a mascara; any mascara will do, apparently (I'll have a word with her about that!). In fact, it was Rosie who introduced me to Benefit by way of these two products, when we were just 18. So, when writing this section of the book, I asked Rosie to bring round her make-up bag, and to my surprise, Rosie had the three products I mentioned above plus – are you ready for this? – one foundation, two concealers, two lipsticks, three lip glosses, two blushers, two highlighters, one eyeshadow palette, two more mascaras and the kitchen sink! Okay, maybe not the sink – that would be ridiculous, right? This, ladies, is a very common scenario that many of us find ourselves in. Opposite, I explain exactly what you need to carry around with you every day. Obviously, what you keep at home is up to you! In fact, I dare you to take a pic with the products you use every day in your hands and the rest of the products left in your make-up bags and tweet or Instagram with #EasyOnTheEyes. I'd love to see your make-up stashes!

Of everything you keep at home, these are the seven products I always have in my handbag. And three of them can be used for more than one thing. Work out which products work best for you and get them in your bag now!

Make-up bag essentials

Base

Don't carry your full foundation around with you. Instead, decant a bit of your base into a clear plastic pot. If you have oily skin, do the same with your favourite powder.

Bronzer

Buy one that comes with a brush and a mirror so that you don't have to carry these separately. Remember, you can use bronzer all over the face, on the eyelids and even on lips.

Colour

Choose either a lipstick, a lip and cheek stain or a cream blush (just the one, ladies – I know it's tempting to pack all three!). You can use these on the cheeks and lips and with just one product the colour will match perfectly!

Eyes

There are some amazing eye-shadow palettes out there, but I prefer to keep these at home. Instead, I carry around a couple of different coloured liners. There are loads of graphic and smoky looks you can create with liner.

Mascara

If you apply mascara in the morning, then you shouldn't really need to top it up throughout the day. However, if you're a mascara junkie like me, then you won't feel safe leaving the house without your magic wand! If you do, you can freshen up your mascara by rubbing a touch of lip balm over the top for a glossy finish.

Brows

As with mascara, your brows should stay put all day if you do them before you leave the house. However, a brow fibre/fiber gel is the perfect product to add colour and to keep those brows in place throughout the day.

Lips

My lips get super-dry, so I always carry a lip balm around with me, although it's usually in my pocket rather than in my make-up bag. Balms also add a glossy finish, so you can use them over lipstick, too.

So these are your make-up bag essentials. Your bag's going to feel twice as light now!

Now I know I said seven things, but this one isn't for your face: a perfume sample. Whenever I buy my full-size fragrance, I always ask for a sample too. Most retailers stock these and they are great to keep in your make-up bag for an afternoon spritz.

Brows

Someone once told me that if you have nice eyebrows you literally have everything you need in life! Okay, so this might be slightly dramatic (shoes are obviously more important!), but when it comes to your face, a good brow makes all the difference. Until Cara Delevingne came along, no one really spoke about eyebrows, and then BAM! Brow-mania! And rightly so, I'd say.

Your eyebrows are so important. Good brows are like an instant eyelift: they make you look younger, more awake and well groomed. Whether you have tons of brow hair, or hardly any, there is a brow solution out there for you.

Remember, your brows are sisters, not twins!

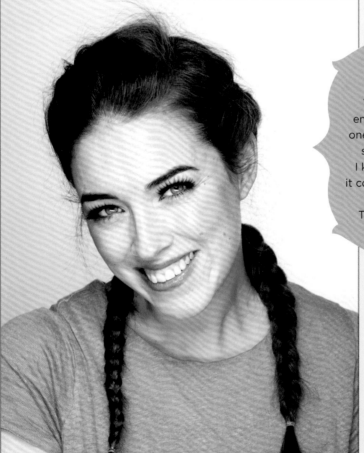

Ask the expert

Visiting a brow bar is the best way to ensure really great brows. It can take just one wrongly tweezed brow hair to ruin the shape, so leave it to the brow experts. I know I may be a little biased, but when it comes to brow shaping, I honestly believe Benefit are the best in the business. They've been waxing brows since 1976!

Map your brows

This is a great thing to do at home when applying your product to keep the perfect brow shape between waxes. At Benefit your brows are mapped first to ensure you get the perfect shape for you. Here's how to do it at home...

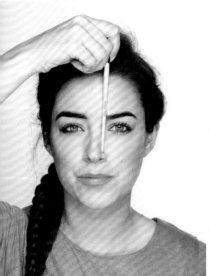 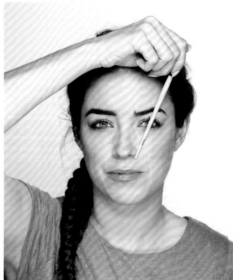 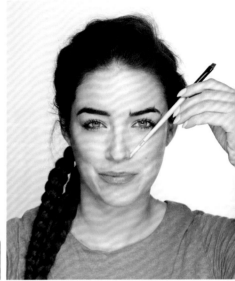

Step 1

Look straight ahead into a mirror. Hold a make-up brush at the dimple of your nose straight up to your brow. Mark with a line using a brow pencil or powder that suits your colouring. Starting here will give a slimming effect to your nose and balance your eyes.

Step 2

Next, hold the brush at the edge of your nose straight through the pupil of your eye to find the arch point. Mark with a line. Draw between the first and second marks and fill in the eyebrow to the arch point using your favourite brow product for an instant eye lift.

Step 3

Move the brush so that it runs from the edge of your nose through the outer corner of the eye and up to the brow. Mark this point to end your brows. As before, draw between this and the arch point, filling in the brow. Ending here will have an eye-opening effect. Wipe away the markers and there you have it, perfectly mapped brows!

You can maintain your brows between waxes using the shape you've created as a guide for tweezing following the instructions on pages 30–31. Remove any stray brow hairs outside the pencilled brow but not any that are too close.

Brow treatments

Need to know more about brows? Well, here it is, the best of the rest on all things eyebrow: the upkeep, choosing the right colour and product, and enhancing them with some simple tips and tricks of the trade.

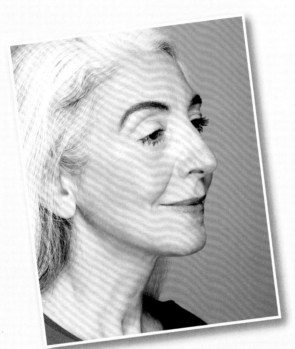

As we get older we tend to loose the tail of the brow. Following the brow-mapping technique on page 29 and using a brow powder to lengthen the brow will open your eyes instantly.

Colour clash
I heart dark brows with blonde hair. Don't be afraid to give dark brows a go, even if you're fair.

Tinting your brows
It only takes 180 seconds to tint your brows and *wow*, what a difference it makes! A brow tint makes your brows look thicker and fuller instantly. Whether you have dark brows, fair brows or even a few silver strands, a brow tint will define and cover, and last for up to 6 weeks! If you're having your brows waxed or threaded, make sure you don't leave without a tint. You can thank me later!

Waxing or threading?
Well, it's completely up to you. Both are good. Personally, I prefer waxing, but that's only because threading is so quick that it scares me – ha! If you're a brow newbie, I would definitely try waxing before threading.

Tweezing
We can't all visit a brow bar every 4–6 weeks. My brows grow nearly as quickly as Usain Bolt

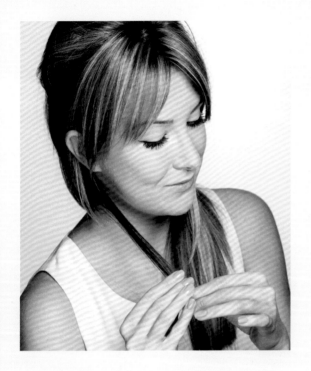

Brow pencils are soft and give you a really natural finish. So they're great if you just have a couple of gaps to fill in. Apply in small strokes through the brow. Using a clean mascara wand (you can buy these in packs from any chemist), brush through the brow to blend in the pencil.

Brow powder and wax: I've put these two together as they tend to come in a little set. The powder adds the colour and the wax keeps the hair in place. This is great if you want a slightly bolder brow. Following the instructions on page 29, mark your points with the powder and then join the dots! Next, mix the powder and wax together with a hard-angled brush, draw against the direction of the hair of your brow in small strokes, then go back with the hair. Repeat until you have the depth and shape that you like.

A simple line of **brow highlighter** under the brow can lift and open your eyes. This one's for everyone. Just draw a line under your brow arch and blend with your fingertips! Done.

doing the 100 metres, so, if you're like me, tweezing can be essential, but can easily go wrong. Just remember these three things:
• Make sure your tweezers are sharp. I love Tweezerman tweezers, as you can send them off to be sharpened for free!
• Always tweeze in the direction of the hair growth. This will ensure you don't snap the hair off, leaving you with a potential ingrown hair!
• Tweeze around the shape of the brow, avoiding the actual shape, as one wrong tweezed hair can ruin your whole brow shape.

Brow products

Yes, brow products! I LOVE YOU!!! Thick brows aren't just for those born with a naturally perfect pair. Brow products can work wonders, especially if your brows have been over-tweezed or if they just don't tend to grow. From waxes to powders, pencils to gels, it's hard to know what products are right for you, so here are a few pointers. First, pick a colour that matches a strand of hair from the base of your hairline.

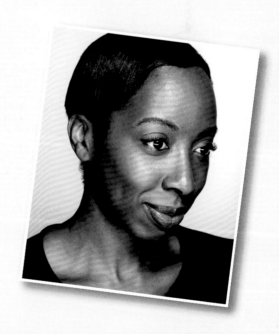

Groom your brows

My brows are like wild animals. I think they're perfect, then I take a selfie and, lo and behold, there's a brow hair out of place. Well, if I haven't applied a clear brow gel, that is! These are literally hair gel for your brows. Genius! Use them on their own, or over the top of any of other product. Just brush them through your brow in the direction of the hair growth and you'll never have a brow drama again.

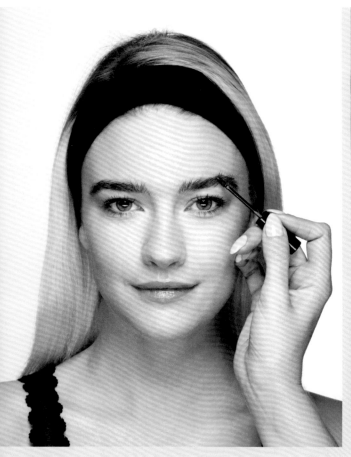

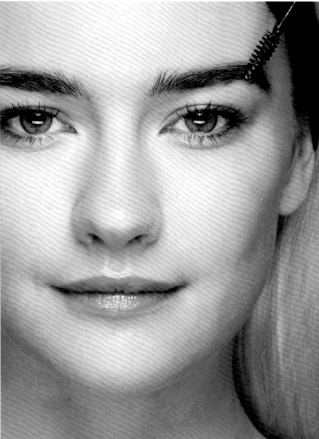

Step 1

If you're short of time then brush-on fibre/fiber gels are amazing for mimicking the appearance of real hair. Benefit's Gimme Brow is my absolute fave! It adds volume to your brows in seconds. To apply, go against the direction of the hair (like back-combing for your brows).

Step 2

Next, follow the brow hairs in the direction of the growth.

Repeat these steps a couple of times for extra drama and depth of colour, and there you have it, instant brow wow!

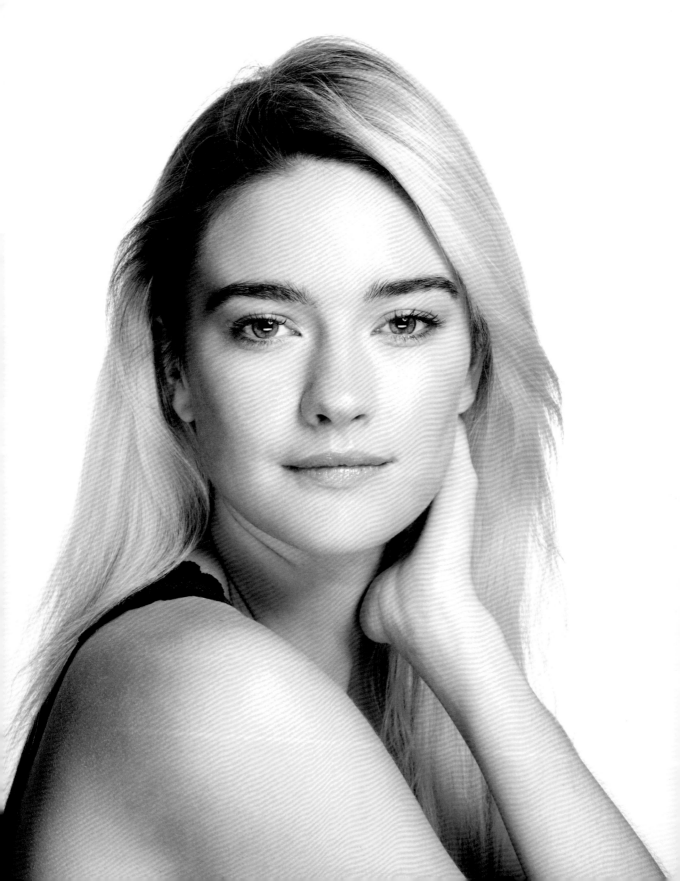

Eye say: play with colour

My absolute favourite thing about make-up is colour! I love to experiment with all different types of shades and tones, but one question I get asked regularly by my clients is 'what colours should I use?' Well, ladies, I say try it all! That's right, if you like the look of a colour, give it a go. As I said earlier, it's only make-up, so you can always take it off if you don't like the look you've created.

However, if you're just starting out with colour, I've created an at-a-glance eye chart below to show you which colours will complement the colour of your eyes.

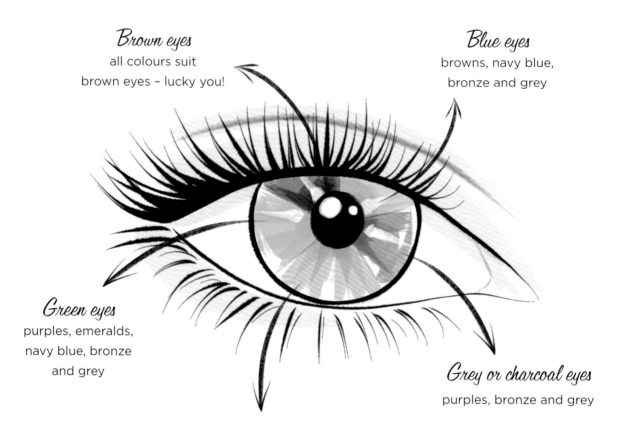

Brown eyes
all colours suit
brown eyes – lucky you!

Blue eyes
browns, navy blue,
bronze and grey

Green eyes
purples, emeralds,
navy blue, bronze
and grey

Grey or charcoal eyes
purples, bronze and grey

Hazel eyes
browns, bronze, purple
and grey

Eye say: the eyes have it

Our eyes are all different shapes and sizes, and all completely stunning. No matter what your eye shape, you can recreate all of the looks within this book as well as develop your own dazzling creations. There are some simple tricks that help when applying make-up on different shapes of eyes so I've written these top tips for you to refer to as you experiment. I just love painting around peepers.

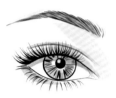 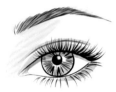

Almond eyes make the most of rich colours and buff eye shadow for longer on almond-shaped eyes.

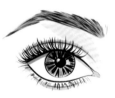

Round eyes elongate the width of the eyes with liner looks like The big flick on pages 114–117.

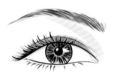 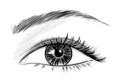

Downturned eyes widen the eyes by focussing on the outer corners with a classic flick (pages 104–109).

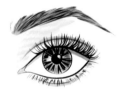

Asian eyes use eye shadow or bronzer to contour the eyelids following the steps on pages 44–45.

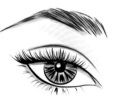 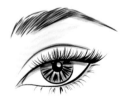

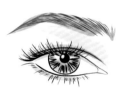 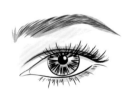

Hooded eyes use matte eye shadows rather than ones with shimmer which might crease.

Applying mascara

Dear mascara, what would we do without you? Thank you for adding length, volume, colour and curl to our feeble lashes. Love every make-up-loving woman in the world, ever! xx

Mascara is definitely my desert-island product. I feel like I look tired and less like me without luscious lashes. You can pick any colour that you like, but the old fave is always going to be black! There's nothing better to define your eyes. Here are my top tips on how to use our old friend.

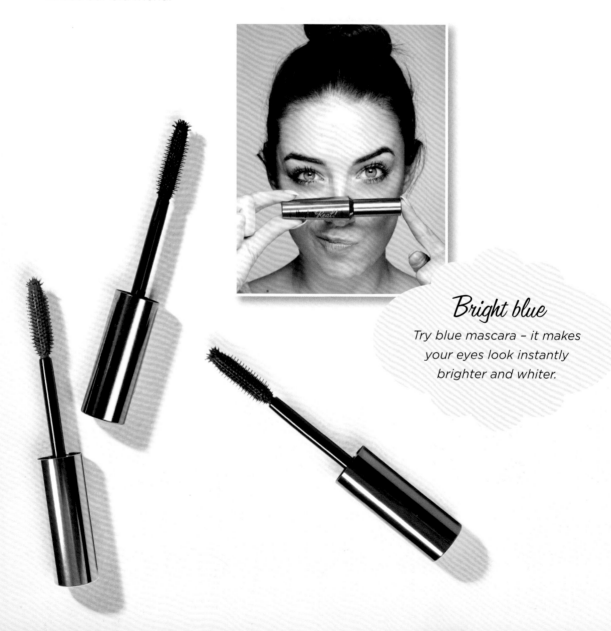

Bright blue

Try blue mascara – it makes your eyes look instantly brighter and whiter.

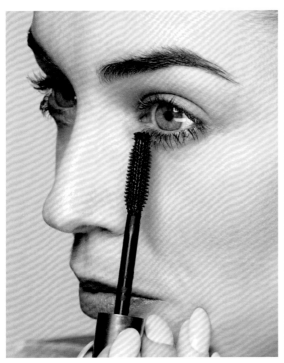

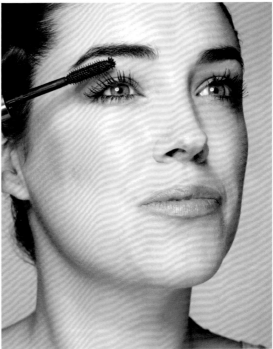

Step 1

Always start with the bottom lashes. If you do the top first, you'll look up to do your bottom and lashes and ruin your eye make-up while the top is still wet! Coat the bottom lashes by holding the wand parallel to the lash line, then hold it vertically and lightly brush onto the lash hair.

Step 2

Coat the top lashes by holding the wand parallel to the lash line and brushing on the mascara. Wiggling it back and forth from the roots will give extra lift.

Step 3

Turn the wand and GO VERTICAL! Use the tip of the wand to apply mascara to any hard-to-reach lashes. This will ensure you catch every single tiny lash and give as much length to your lashes as possible. Pay extra attention to your outer-corner lashes, as the longer these are, the bigger your eyes will look. While the mascara is still slightly wet, apply a second coat for extra oomph!

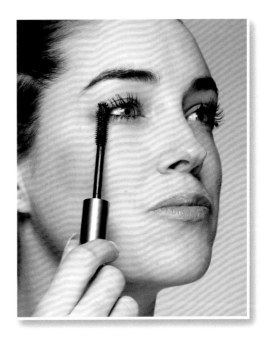

Applying strip eyelashes

False eyelashes look amazing and can really complete a look. However, they can be quite intimidating, as they can be a right pain to apply... until now! Below are my fail-safe, you-just-can't-go-wrong instructions for applying falsies, so give it a go. Remember to always apply your lashes after you have completed your eye make-up. If you put them on first, you'll end up with make-up all over them, which will spoil their effect.

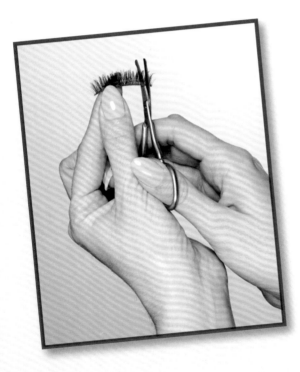

Step 1

Choose the pair of lashes you want to wear, measure the lash against your eye and trim them to the same length as your lash line. Trim from the inner corner so that you do not lose the flick of the lash.

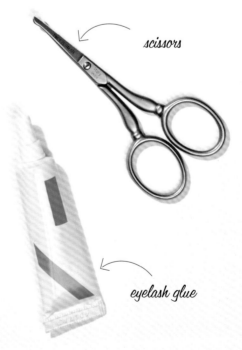

scissors

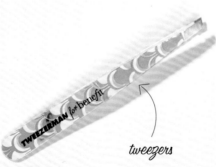

tweezers

eyelash glue

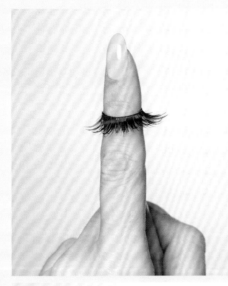

Step 2

Bend the lash around your finger for 30 seconds – this may look strange (no one wants a hairy finger – ha!), but it's vital, as it adds curvature to the lash, meaning that it will sit better on your eye.

Step 3

Now to add the glue. Less is more here, but you do want to add a touch extra on each of the ends. You can apply it straight from the tube, but I like to apply the glue using the end of a cotton bud/swab. Wait a good 30 seconds before applying the lash to your eyes so that the glue is tacky but not wet. To speed up the process, do what I like to call the 'lash dance' (i.e. shake the lash back and forth whilst dancing to your favourite song, but whatever you do, DON'T LET GO!).

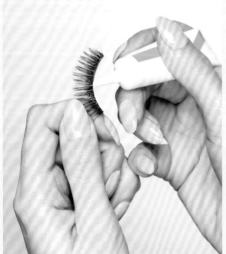

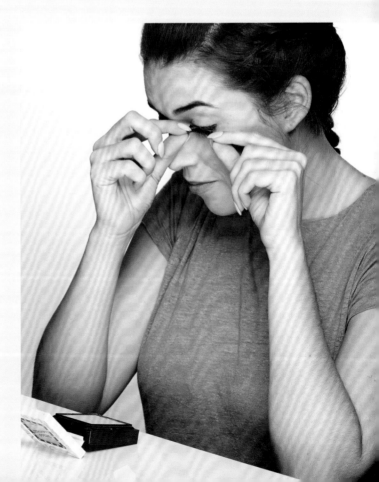

Step 4

Put a mirror flat on a table and look down into it. This will help you to apply the lash super-close to the lash line. Don't worry if it's not quite perfect, because you still have time to move the lash.

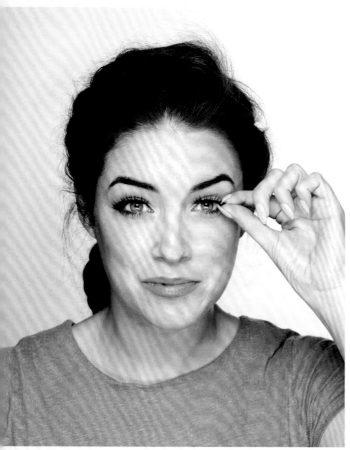

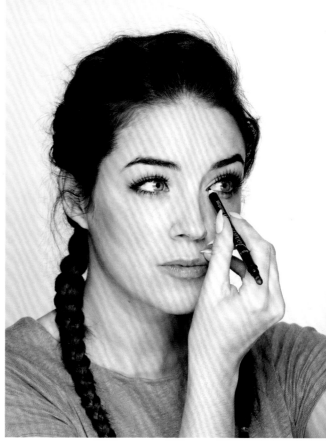

Step 5

Squeeze the false lashes and your natural lashes together with your fingers. This will mean that there's no horrible gap between the two.

Step 6

Finally, to make it look more seamless, add black eyeliner to the gap between the inner corner of your eye and the beginning of the false lash. Et voilà! You are now a lash pro!

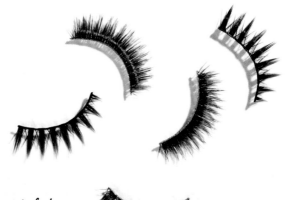

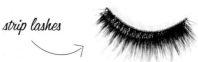

strip lashes

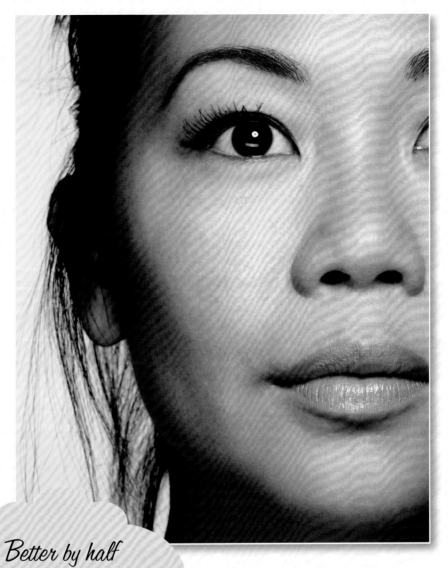

Better by half

Apply half-lashes in the same way as strip lashes for a more natural-looking flick.

Step 1

Either buy a pair of half-lashes or choose a pair of full lashes, measure the lash against your eye and cut at the halfway point from the inner corner so that you don't lose the flick of the lash.

Step 2

Apply the half-lash at the outer corner of the eye following steps 3–6 on pages 39–40.

Applying cluster eyelashes

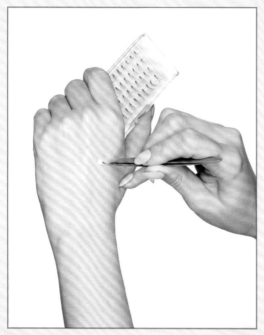

Sometimes you want to give your lashes an extra boost – cluster lashes are great for this. They are sets of three to four individual lashes bonded together and can last two to three days if you look after them. Be warned though, these beauties can be addictive!

Step 1
Start with clean lashes and apply your eye make-up. Don't apply your mascara yet. Put a tiny drop of lash glue on the back of your hand. Pick up a lash cluster using slant-edge tweezers, gripping the cluster close to the base, not by the tip, which could tear the lashes. Dip the base into the glue. Wait about 15 seconds to give the glue time to get sticky before you apply it.

Step 2
Tilt your head back so you can see your lash line in the mirror. Starting at the outer corner of your eye, stick the cluster in the first open spot you see between your lashes, wiggling it in so it sits right on the lash line, not above it. Working inward, add a few more clusters on any open spots. About six sets should be enough for one eye.

Step 3
When you've finished both eyes, leave your lashes alone for five minutes to let the glue dry, then gently sweep with mascara.

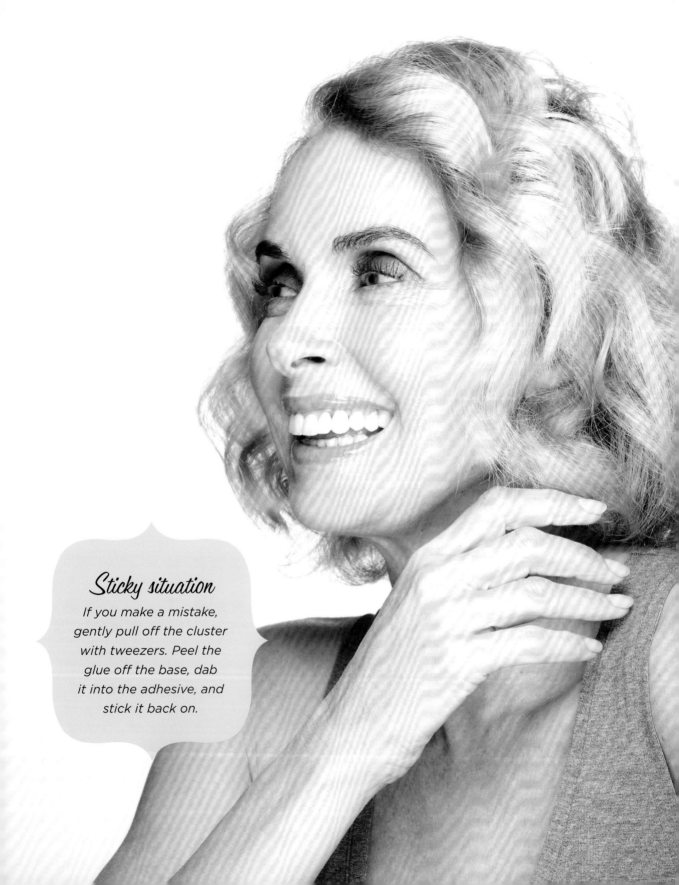

Sticky situation

If you make a mistake, gently pull off the cluster with tweezers. Peel the glue off the base, dab it into the adhesive, and stick it back on.

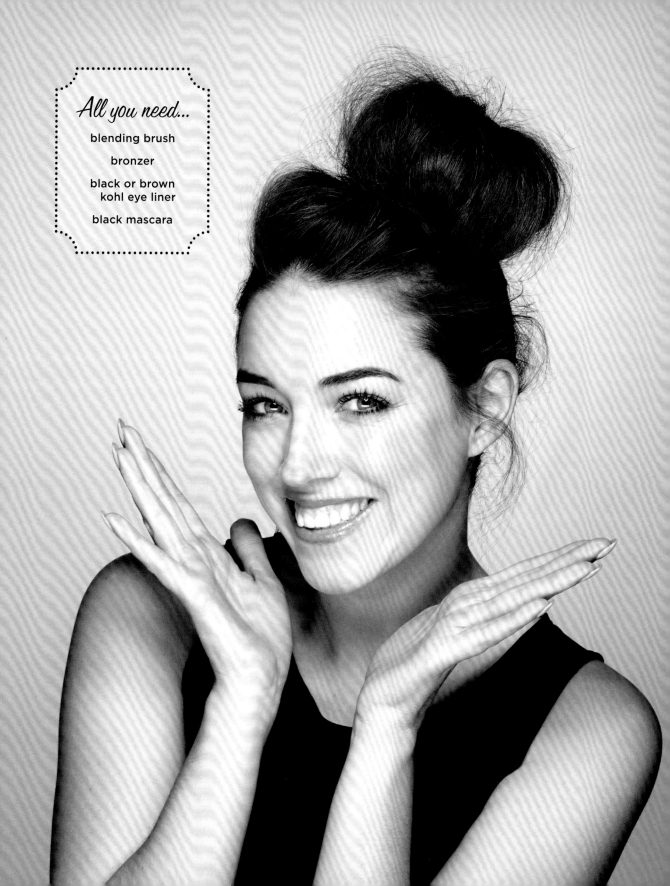

My everyday eye look in 5 minutes

So, we all have those things that we go to when we can't make a decision. Our 'go-to' outfit, our 'go-to' dinner and our 'go-to' TV programme. Our make-up is no exception. If there's one 'go-to' eye look that I wear 80 per cent of the time, then it's a contoured eye with an under-eye liner flick. It's easy to wear and it only takes 5 minutes!

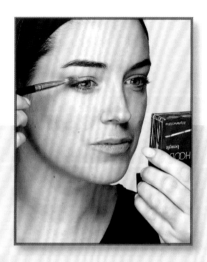

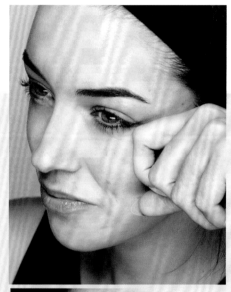

Step 1

Contouring is not just for your face! Contouring your eyes is so simple to do, and it adds definition and warmth instantly. Take your bronzer (I prefer a matte bronzer for a natural finish) and sweep it over the eyelid and into the socket using a blending brush. Done!

Step 2

Take a kohl liner, apply it under your lower lashes and use the knuckle from your index finger to sweep it up towards the angle of your brow. This is the easiest eyeliner flick you'll ever do!

Step 3

Add tonnes of mascara (see pages 36–37). Yep, that's it – super quick and simple! Hopefully one of the looks in this book will become your 'go-to' look. Tweet or Instagram me (@Lisa_Benefit) with #EasyOnTheEyes.

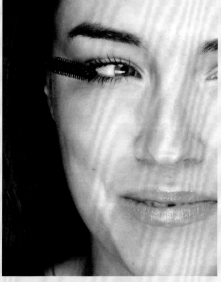

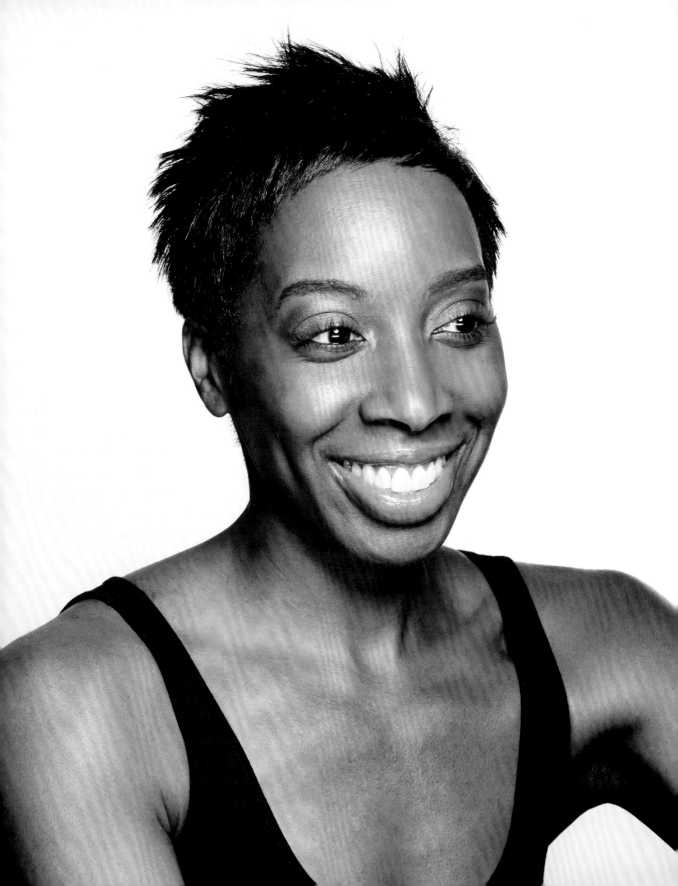

Smokin' eyes

Are you ready to get smoky, ladies? Well, this chapter is most certainly going to help you do that! Smoky eyes look really beautiful when done properly. And I'm going to show you how to create the perfect smoky eye whether you've got 5, 15 or 30 minutes.

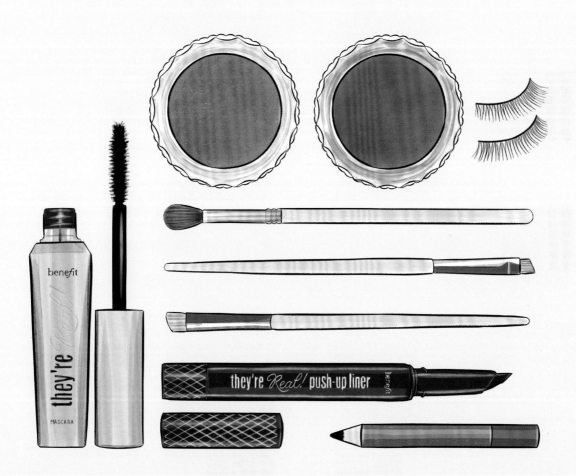

Classic smoky eye in 5 minutes

A smoky eye in 5 minutes. Impossible, I hear you say! Well, fear not, ladies, I'm going to show you how to achieve this look in the same amount of time that it takes you to make a cuppa!

Pick your eye shadow, just the one. I prefer powder shadows for this look, as they are easy to build and blend, but colourwise, it's up to you! I've chosen a dark grey, as it's the shade associated most with a classic smoke.

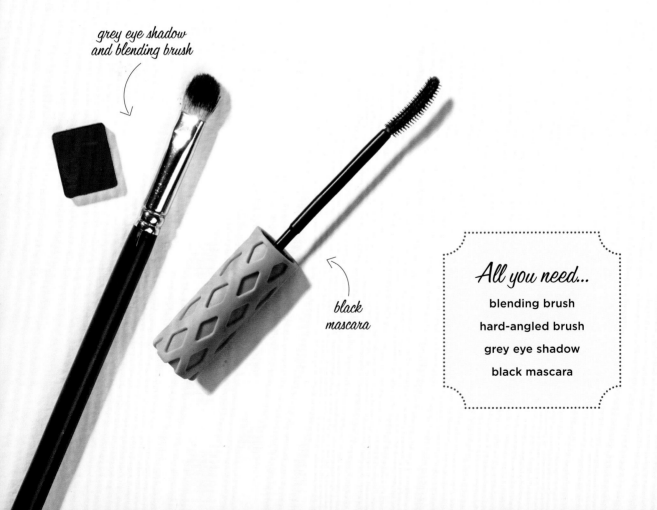

grey eye shadow and blending brush

black mascara

All you need...

blending brush

hard-angled brush

grey eye shadow

black mascara

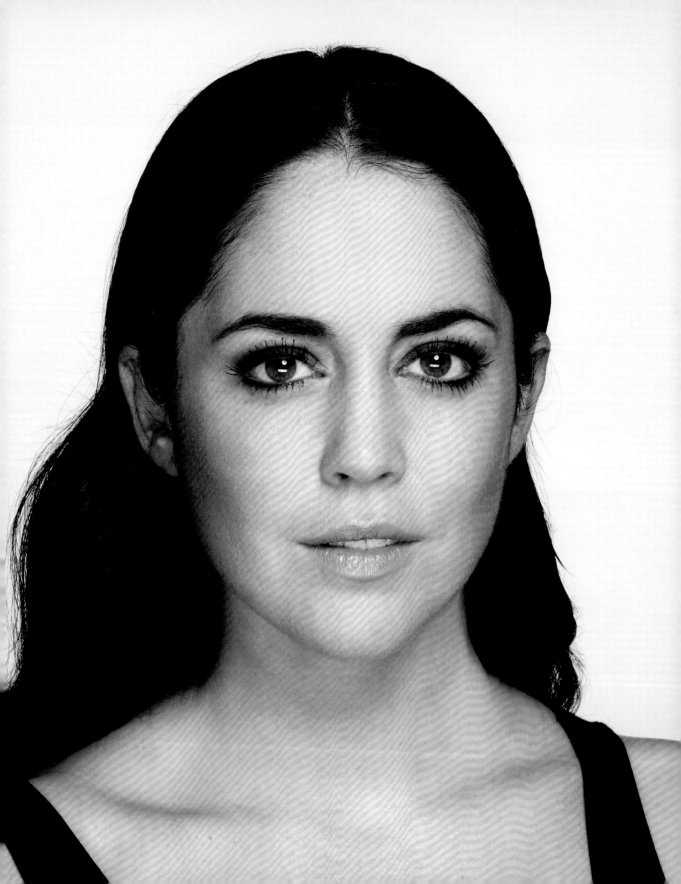

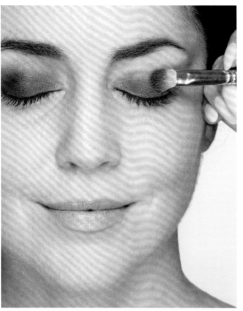

Step 1

Take a blending brush and apply your eye shadow to the centre of your eyelid. Using the same brush, blend the shadow backwards and forwards across the eyelid. If you find it easier, keep your eyes open for this. Take the shadow into the socket, but don't take it any higher. Also, don't take it any further out than the angle from the corner of your eye to the corner of your brow. Blend in circular motions to get an airbrushed finish. You can add as many layers of the shadow as you like. The more you add, the darker the look. Take your time to build the colour up, but not too long, as you only have 5 minutes!

Step 2

If you want to make the look a bit more dramatic, apply the same shadow under the lower lash line using a hard-angled brush for precision.

Step 3

Add lashings of mascara, bottom lashes first. See pages 36–37. And that's it, three steps! That's 100 seconds per step – easy!! 3, 2, 1, GO!

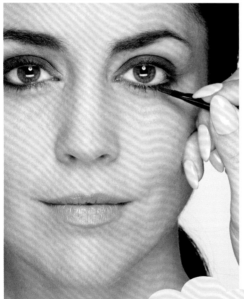

Keep it clean

A nude lip looks beautiful with this look, just pat a little concealer onto your lips for a naked finish.

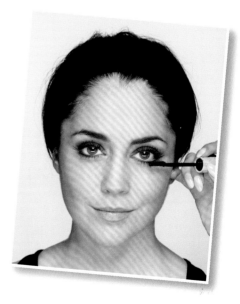

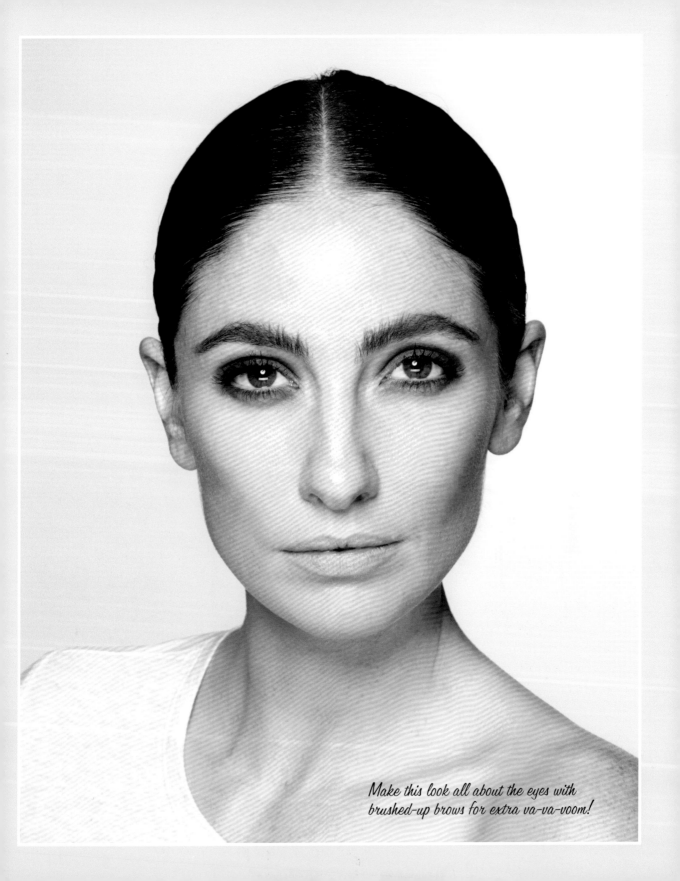

Make this look all about the eyes with brushed-up brows for extra va-va-voom!

Bronze smoky eye in 5 minutes

Bronze-toned eye shadows are the queens of the shadow land, as they pretty much suit everyone. Yay!

Bronzes are usually metallic-based shadows, which really brighten the eye. The lighter the bronze shade you pick, the more natural the look. Pick a colour you like, but for the look below, I'm using a rich bronze for the main shadow and a deep bronze for under the lash line.

Midtown mid-tones

If you have hooded eyes (see page 35), avoid very dark colours that make your eyes look heavy and stick to mid-tones.

All you need...

blending brush

cotton bud/swab
or hard-angled brush

pencil brush

bronze eye shadow

black or brown liquid
or gel eye liner

black or brown
mascara

black mascara

bronze
eye shadow

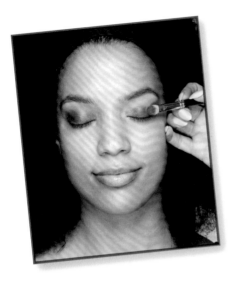

Step 1

Start in the centre of the eye and apply the rich bronze shadow using a fluffly blending brush. Blend the shadow back and forth over the lid. Go into the socket, but don't go any higher. Blend in circular motions to build up the depth of colour. Repeat this a couple of times to build up an even layer of shadow.

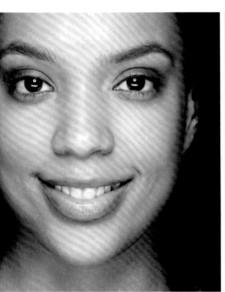

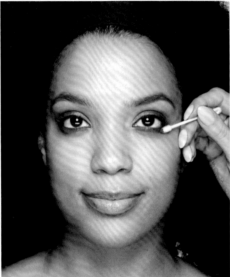

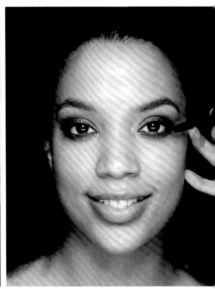

Step 2

I love a bit of liner with a bronze smoky eye. Apply a Fine and defined line following the instructions on pages 90–93, using a black or brown liquid or gel liner.

Step 3

Using a cotton bud/swab or hard-angled brush, press the deep bronze shadow under the lower lash line. Blend with a pencil brush to soften the edges. This will really define the eye.

Step 4

Add lashings of mascara, bottom lashes first (see pages 36–37). Beautiful bronze smoky eye quickly completed!

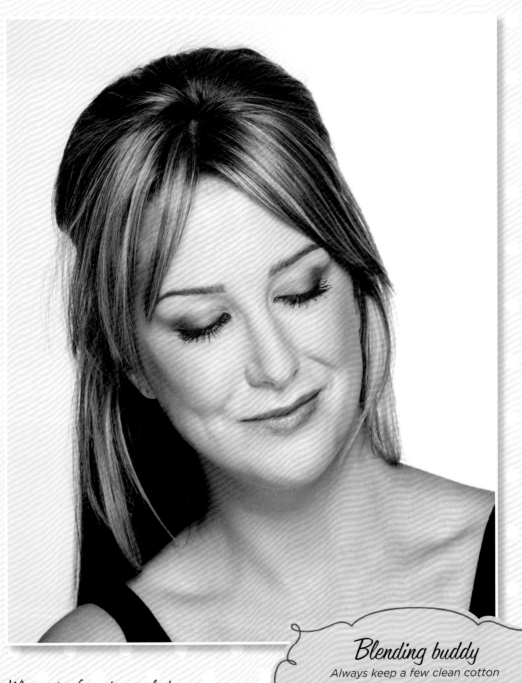

When going for a bronze look, warm up your complexion with a touch of bronzer on the cheeks as well.

Blending buddy

Always keep a few clean cotton buds/swabs in your make-up bag, as they're super handy for blending.

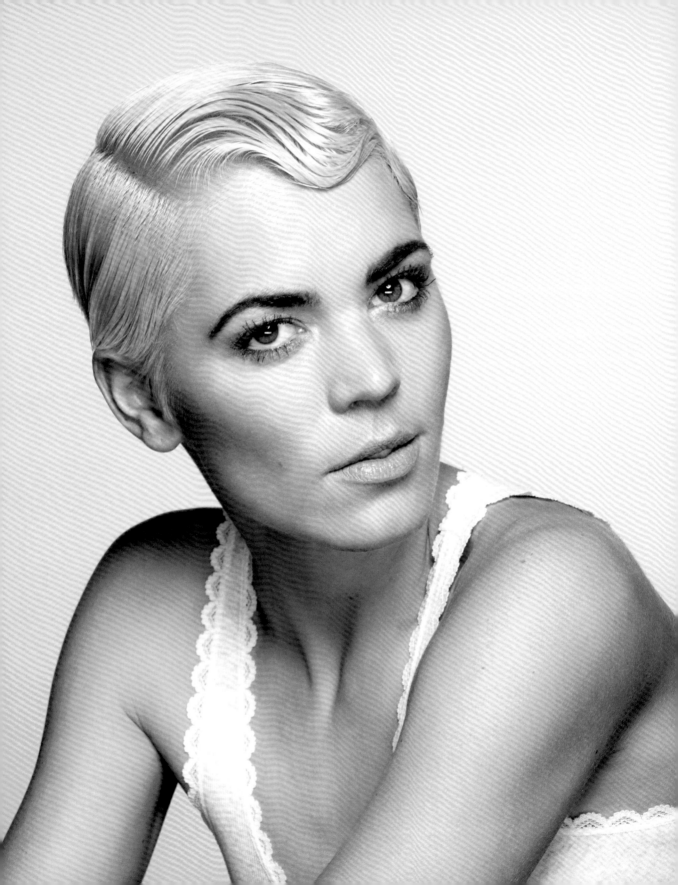

Colourful smoky eye in 5 minutes

I love experimenting with different colours. A colourful smoky eye can be super-quick, but gives your whole look a real pop! If you're not sure what colours suit you, then refer to my colour chart on page 34. This will give you a basic idea, but don't be afraid to give anything a go.

As always, pick your colour. We're only going to use one colour here, so feel free to use a powder or cream eye shadow, whichever you prefer. I'm using a gorgeous pastel purple.

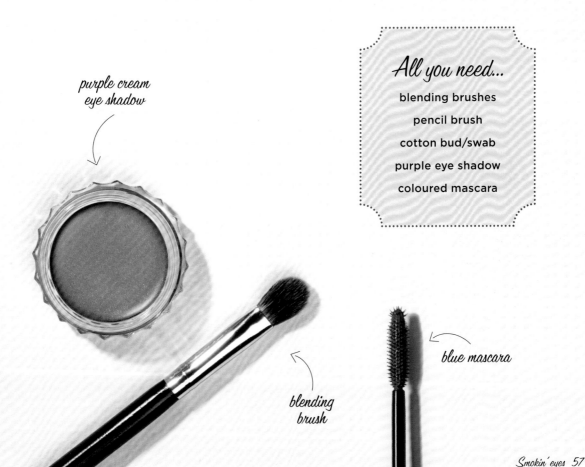

purple cream eye shadow

All you need...
blending brushes
pencil brush
cotton bud/swab
purple eye shadow
coloured mascara

blending brush

blue mascara

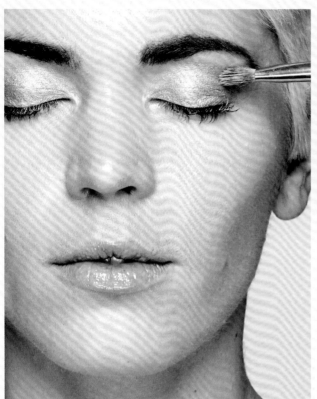

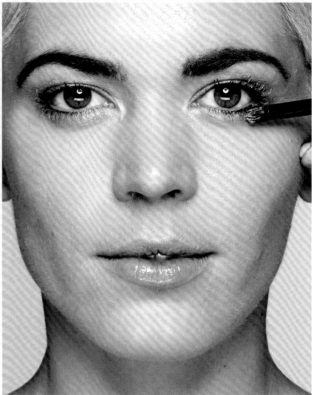

Step 1

Start in the centre of your eyelid and blend the shadow with a blending brush in circular motions all over the eyelid. Go into the socket, but don't go any higher. Take a clean blending brush and blend the shadow again. You want to get the colour as even as possible and using a clean brush will help you achieve this.

Step 2

I love framing the whole eye with colour. Using the same colour and a pencil brush, blend the shadow under the lower lash line into the corner of the eye and connect the outer corner of colour to the upper eyelid.

Rainbow colours

You can use any colour and any type of eye shadow for this look, so really experiment. The more the colours clash, the edgier your look will be.

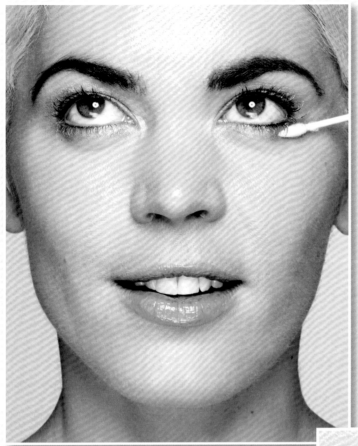

Step 3
Use a cotton bud/swab to soften the edges of the colour.

Step 4
Add tonnes of mascara (see pages 36–37). You could use a matching coloured mascara or a blue mascara (as shown) to really show off the look. Gorgeous!

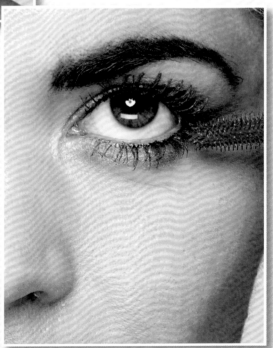

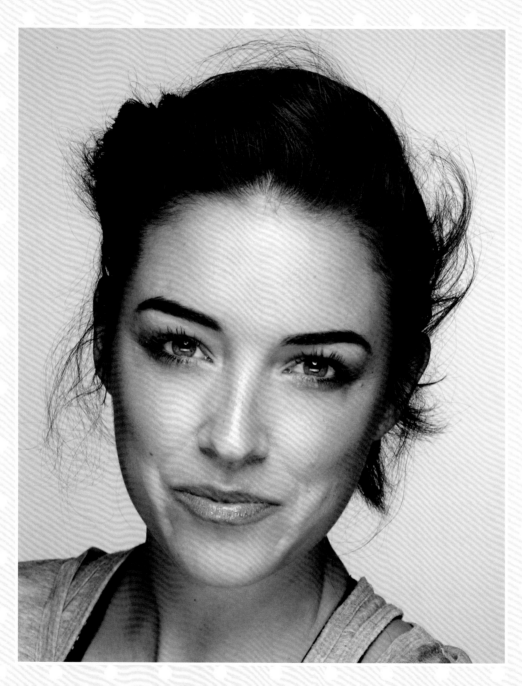

*I love multi-purpose products! It saves
space and money, and you can look good using less.*

Make-up in the wrong places

Nearly all make-up products are multi-use. So don't just think that eye shadow is for your eyes and lipstick is for your lips, make the most of your favourite beauty products by experimenting with some of my top tips.

Easy eyes

• Apply bronzer to eyelids using a blending brush to make your eyes look bigger.
• Lip gloss on your eyelid adds a gorgeous sheen (see pages 130–133), just don't use a gloss that's too sticky!

Colourful cheeks

• Lipstick on your cheeks can be gorgeous, as it gives you a pop of colour with a dewy finish.

Perfect pout

• Concealer on your lips looks fab if you're looking for a nude finish. It's also fab as a primer for your lips if applied before lipstick, as it creates a long-lasting base.
• Using a metallic eye shadow in a soft gold colour in the centre of your lips will give your pout that extra oomph.

Secret slimming

• Apply a matte brown eye shadow down the side of your nose for a slimming effect.
• Using Vaseline jelly down the centre of your nose and on the cheek bones is a great alternative to highlighter. It gives a really fresh finish, perfect in summer, to contour the face.

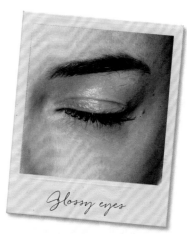

Glossy eyes

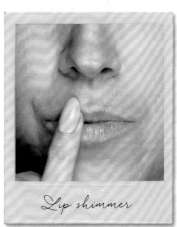

Lip shimmer

Classic smoky eye in 15 minutes

I decided to Google 'things you can achieve in 15 minutes' and it's actually amazing how much you can get done in such a short period of time. I have to say, some of the things were slightly strange, such as 'write your own obituary' or 'do 200 star jumps' – not quite what I had in mind! My faves were 'call someone you haven't spoken to in a while', 'run a mile', and 'eat loads of chocolate' – ha! So, back to the point, a classic smoky eye in 15 minutes will be a doddle.

Pick your eye shadows – you'll need three shades: a pale or nude colour, a light grey and a dark grey.

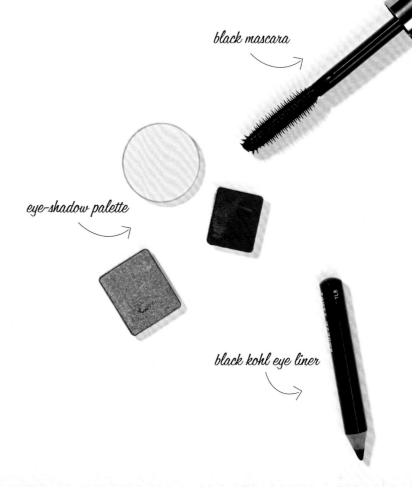

black mascara

All you need...

blending brush

cotton bud/swab or hard-angled brush

three light–dark grey eye shadows (or a 3-colour eye-shadow palette)

black kohl eye liner

white kohl eye liner (optional)

black mascara

eye-shadow palette

black kohl eye liner

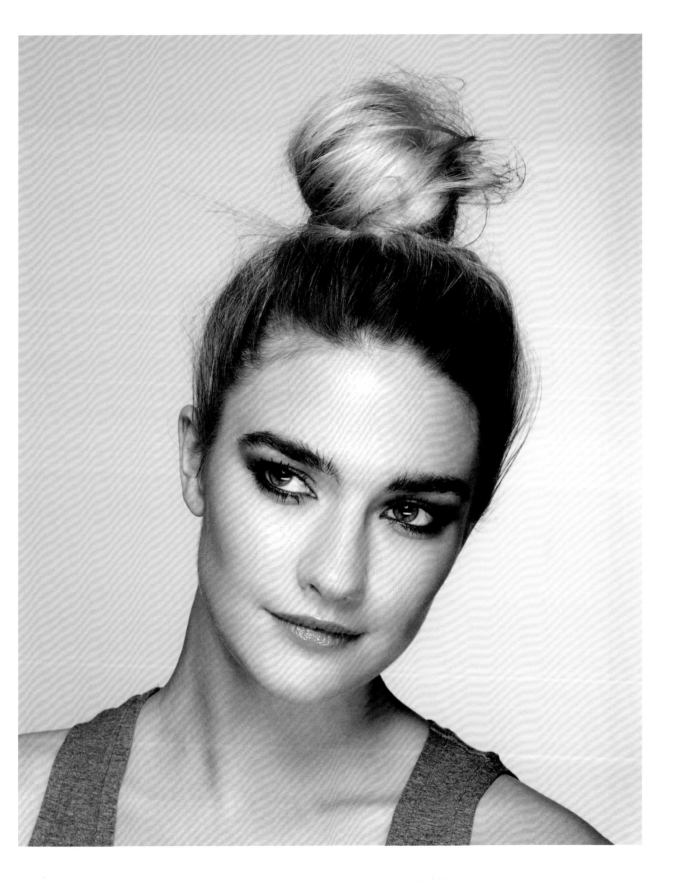

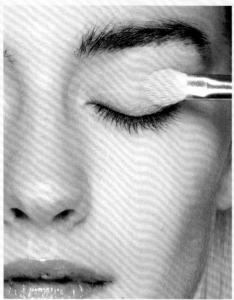

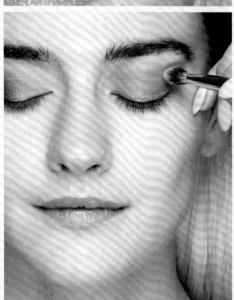

Step 1

Start with the lightest shade and apply it all over your lid with a fluffy blending brush. Remember to go into the socket but not any higher. Take this shade into the corner of the eye, too, as this will brighten the look.

Step 2

Take your medium shade and, using the same brush, apply this into the socket of the eye and halfway along the lid from the outer corner. Take a clean blending brush and blend, blend, blend in circular motions for an airbrushed finish.

Step 3

This step is going to give you that super-classic smoky finish. Take your third and final shade, the darkest of the bunch. Less is more with this one, but don't worry if you make a bit of a mess at first – it's only make-up! With the same brush you've been using to apply your shadow, apply it a third of the way over the lid and into the socket from the outer corner. Blend in circular motions, just like before. You can layer this shade for a darker look if you wish.

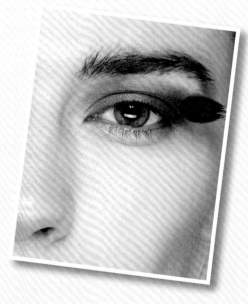

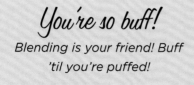

You're so buff!
Blending is your friend! Buff
'til you're puffed!

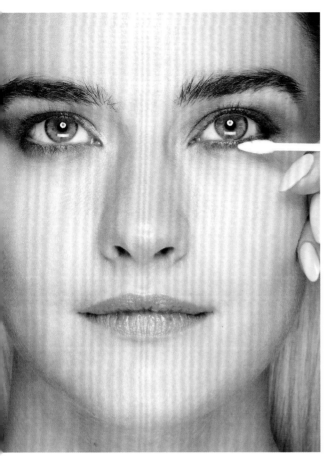
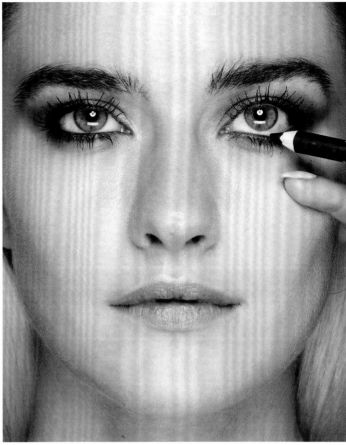

Step 4

Again with the darkest shade, put a little under the lower lash line using a cotton bud/swab or hard-angled brush. This is going to frame the eye beautifully. Blend backwards and forwards with a cotton bud/swab for a soft finish.

Step 5

It's liner time! For this step, you have two options. For a dark, defined finish, use a kohl pencil in the waterline of the eye following the instructions on pages 98–101. If you have small eyes, or you want more of a fresh, bright finish, use a pinky-white pencil in the waterline.

Finish the look by adding tonnes of black mascara (see pages 36–37). Add at least two coats for extra drama.

Now take a look in the mirror and think, 'Yep, I could have run a mile in the last 15 minutes, but I'm glad I chose a classic smoky eye, because look how bloomin' gorgeous I look!'

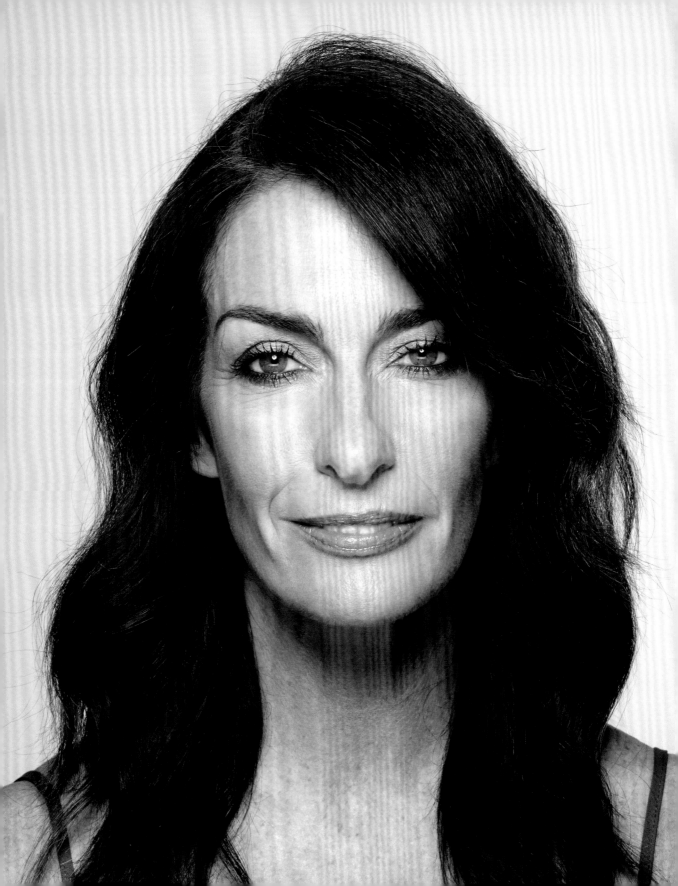

Bronze smoky eye in 15 minutes

Three times longer than a 5-minute look equals three colours instead of one.

This is where readymade eye-colour palettes are fab. They always consist of colours that complement each other, making your colour selection easy.

Pick your eye shadows. You'll need a gold as well as a medium and deep bronze, then we're ready to start.

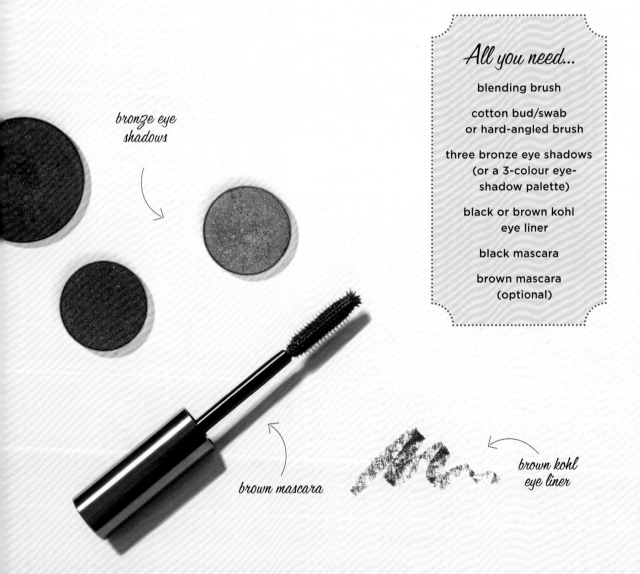

bronze eye shadows

brown mascara

brown kohl eye liner

All you need...

blending brush

cotton bud/swab or hard-angled brush

three bronze eye shadows (or a 3-colour eye-shadow palette)

black or brown kohl eye liner

black mascara

brown mascara (optional)

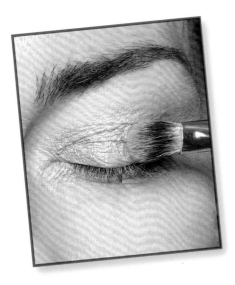

Step 1

Buff the gold shadow onto the lid using a fluffy blending brush. Make sure you don't go any higher than the socket.

Step 2

Next, take your medium bronze shadow. This is going to be used to contour your eyes to give them more definition. The easiest way to do this is by looking straight ahead into a mirror and moving your brush back and forth into the socket of the eye. Keep blending until you get a beautifully even finish.

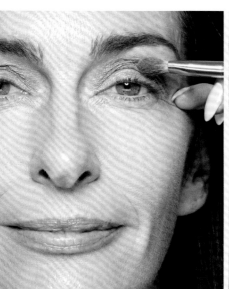
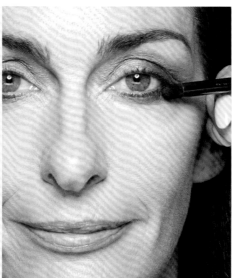
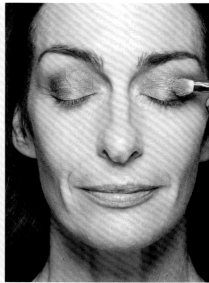

Step 3

Now to smoke it up with the darker shade. A deep bronze shadow looks so beautiful around the eye. This is all about the outer corner of the eye. I like to use a pencil brush to apply the dark shade, as it's important that you don't apply too much. Pat it onto the outer third of the eyelid and then blend, blend, blend!

Using the same brush blend the deep bronze shadow under the lower lash line as well.

Step 4

Next, go back to your gold shadow and pat a small amount into the centre of your eyelid to highlight the round. Blend delicately with a clean blending brush.

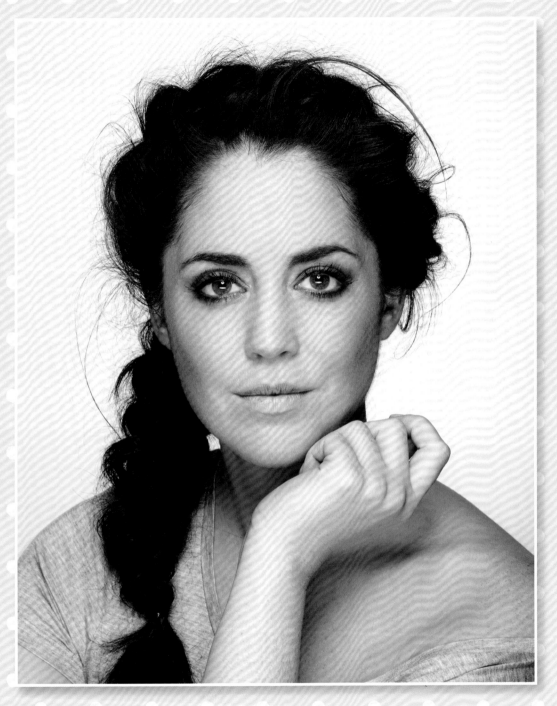

If you have brown eyes, match the dark bronze
shadow to your eye colour for an extra-sultry look.

Colourful smoky eye in 15 minutes

Using jewel-toned eye shadows can look beautiful on the eye.

For this look I've gone for emerald green and navy blue. I'm going to use one tone on the lid and one under the lower lash line. Make sure you do your eyes first when using colour, as you can then just wipe away any excess shadow that drops, rather than worrying about ruining your base.

All you need...

blending brushes

cotton bud/swab

two eye shadows of your choice (or a 2-colour eye-shadow palette)

black kohl eye liner

black mascara

make-up remover

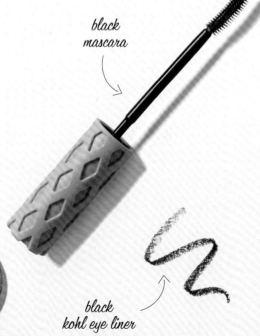

black mascara

green and blue eye shadows

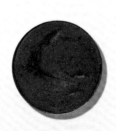

black kohl eye liner

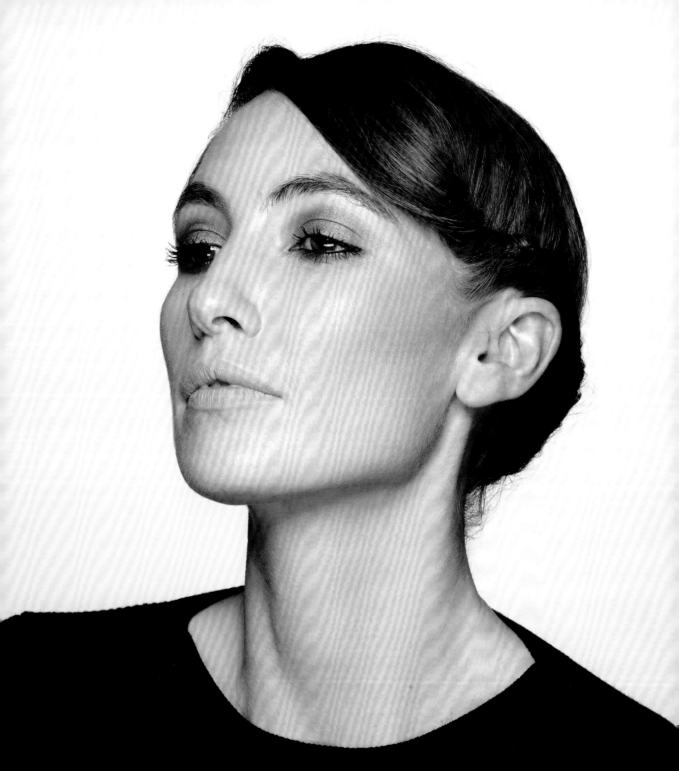

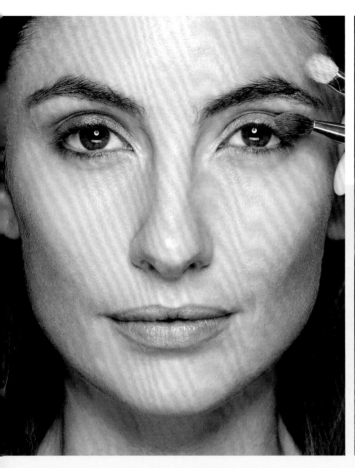
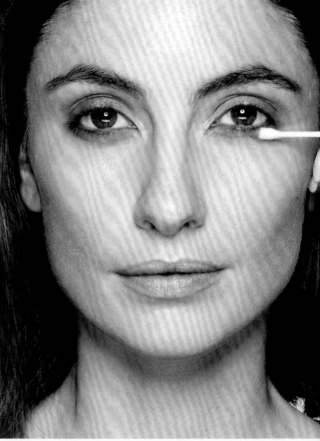

Step 1

Take the green or lighter of your shadows and apply all over the eyelid with a fluffy blending brush. I like to have a clean blending brush on hand to buff when doing this look. The more you buff colour, the better it looks. So don't be afraid to layer and buff, layer and buff. The more you add, the darker the look. Take your time to build it up (but not too long, though, as you only have 15 minutes!).

Step 2

Apply the navy blue or darker of your shadows under the lower lash line. I want this to look vibrant, but soft, so I'm applying and blending with a cotton bud/swab. Cotton buds/swabs are your best friend – they can buff and blend to perfection and they can clean up any mess without ruining a look.

Air-brushes

Clean blending brushes are essential for an airbrush finish. To clean brushes, run them under lukewarm water, lather with a little baby shampoo, then rinse well.

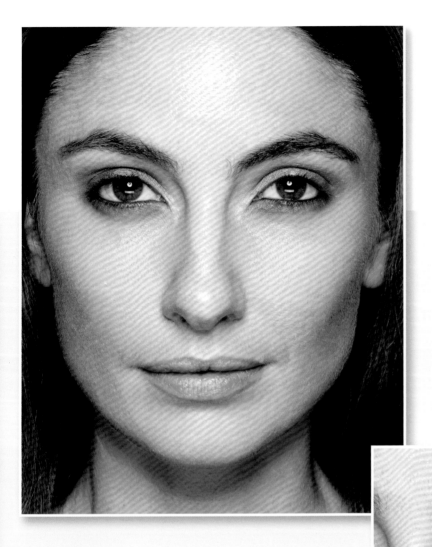

Step 3

I like to add some black liner to this look. Underline the eye with black kohl eye liner and apply it in the waterline following the instructions on pages 98–101. It's super-easy to do and it really pulls a look together.

Step 4

Now, to add mascara. I'm layering those lashes with jet black (see pages 36–37). Bold, bright and beautiful!

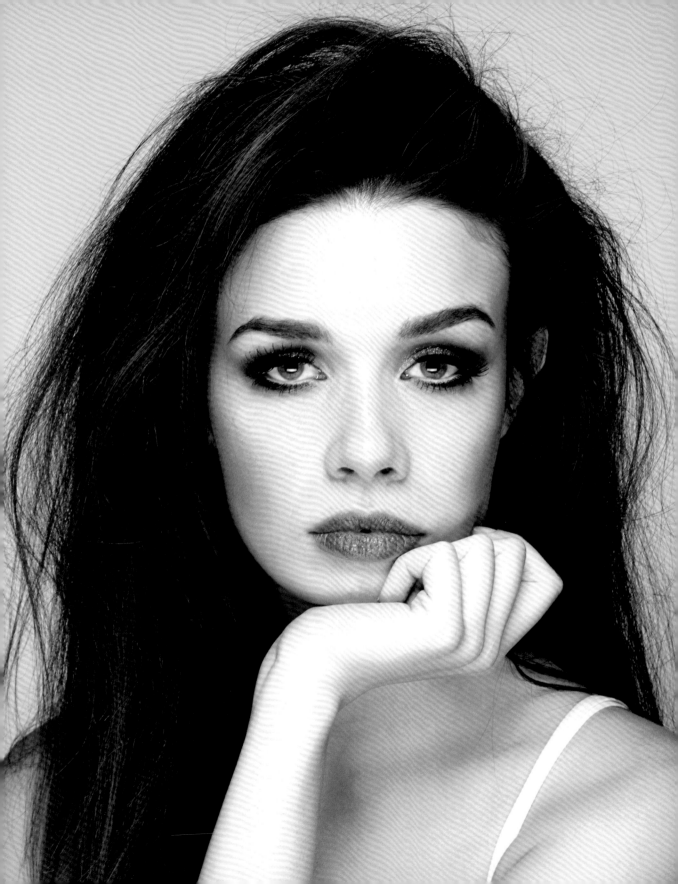

Classic smoky eye in 30 minutes

You've got the time, so let's make you shine with the ultimate smokin' hot eye look!
We're going to use a smoky eye palette again for this classic smoke (as on pages 62–65), but we're going to add a gel eye liner, false eyelashes and a touch of glitter. The glitter's optional, but everyone loves a bit of glitter, right?

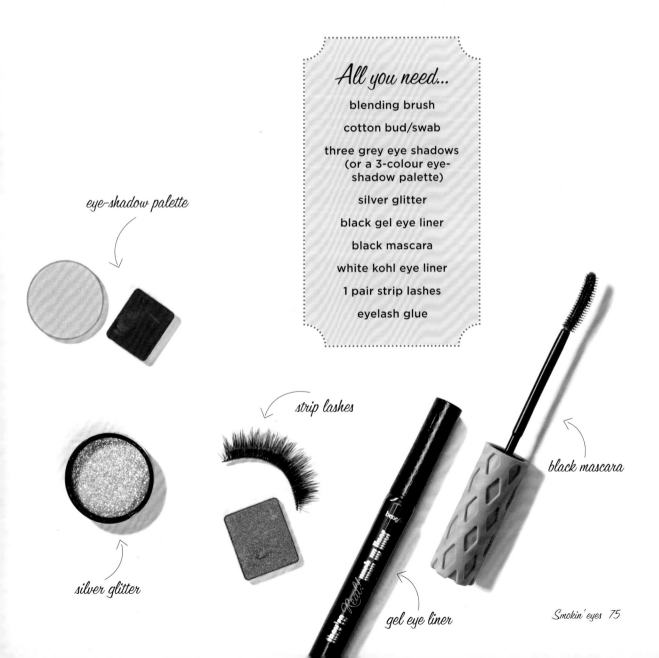

All you need...

blending brush

cotton bud/swab

three grey eye shadows
(or a 3-colour eye-
shadow palette)

silver glitter

black gel eye liner

black mascara

white kohl eye liner

1 pair strip lashes

eyelash glue

eye-shadow palette

strip lashes

black mascara

silver glitter

gel eye liner

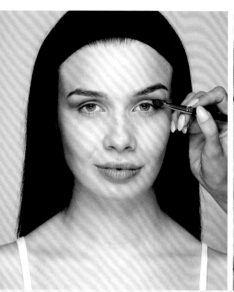
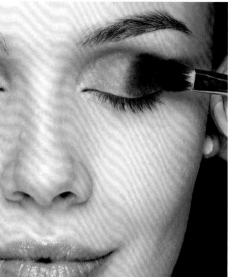
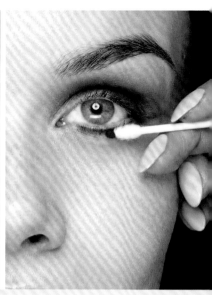

Step 1

Take the lighest shade in the palette and sweep this over your eyelid using a fluffy blending brush, up to the socket of your eye. Blend backwards and forwards for an even base colour. Do the same with the medium shade.

Step 2

It's all about the darkest shade for this look. Apply it in small amounts using the same blending brush on the outer third of the eyelid and build it up. Blend inwards, but don't take it any higher than the socket.

Step 3

Apply the same shade under the lower lash line using a cotton bud/swab.

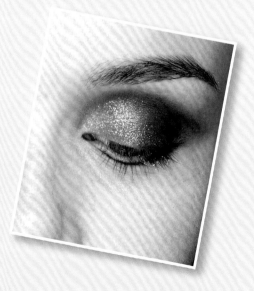

Step 4

I heart anything that shimmers and shines, so I've taken a gorgeous silvery grey glitter and added it to this look. Using your ring finger, pat this into the centre of the lid and towards the inner corner of the eye. This will add instant glamour!

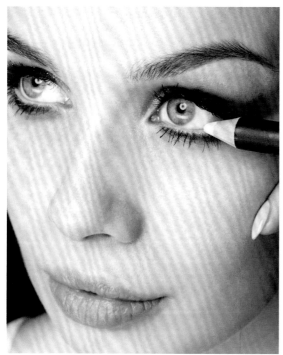
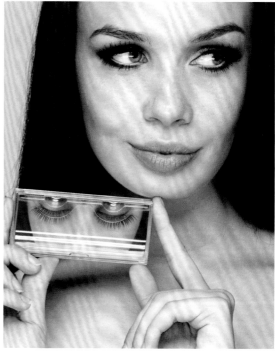

Step 5

Liner? Flick. (See what I did there?) Head to the liner section to master gel liners – choose either the Fine and defined look (pages 90–93) or The classic flick (pages 104–107) to apply black gel eye liner along the top lash line for extra drama. Then apply white kohl eye liner to the waterline following the instructions on pages 98–101.

Step 6

Apply two layers of mascara, starting with the bottom lashes (see pages 36–37), and that's all for the make-up steps.

Step 7

Then, if you're feeling like you want more, add a pair of false eyelashes (see pages 38–43) – it's time to lash it up! I love lashes. They add glamour and drama instantly. They also look incredible in photographs! So, there you have it. The ultimate smokin' hot eye look!

Rose tints

A rose-coloured, matte, stained lip looks great with this look.

Bronze smoky eye in 30 minutes

Bronzes, coppers and golds make for a beautiful sultry look and work well with any eye colour. For this 30-minute look, I'm doing things a bit differently and using masking tape to create the shape of the smoke. So get yourself an eye-shadow palette with the three shades, raid your dad's shed for a roll of masking tape and get ready to wow!

All you need...

masking tape

blending brushes

cotton bud/swab

three bronze eye shadows (or a 3-colour eye-shadow palette)

bronze glitter

black gel eye liner

black mascara

1 pair strip lashes

eyelash glue

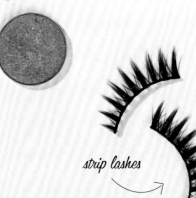

black mascara

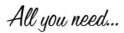

bronze glitter

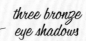

three bronze eye shadows

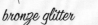

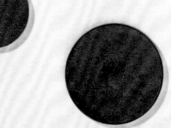

strip lashes

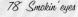

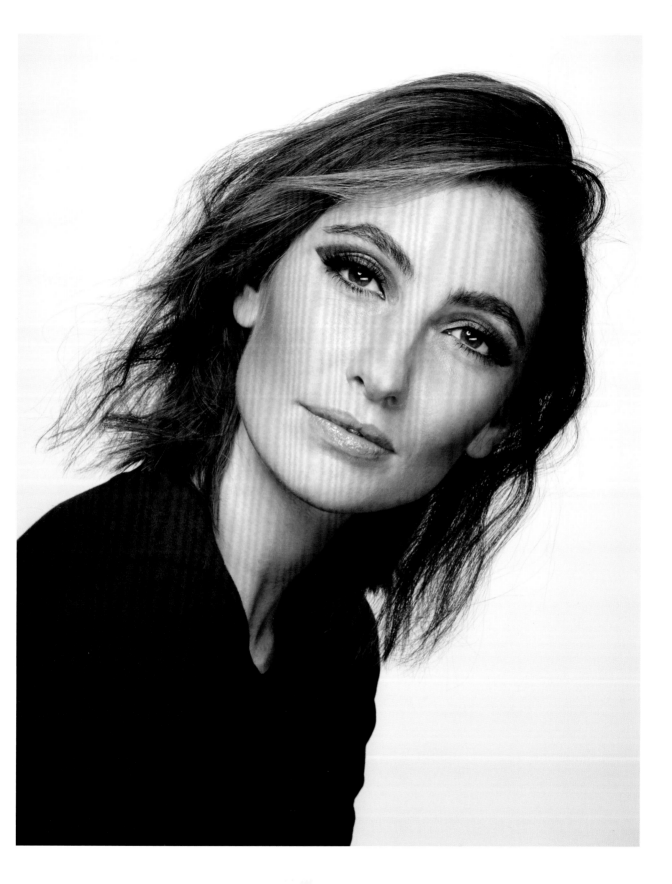

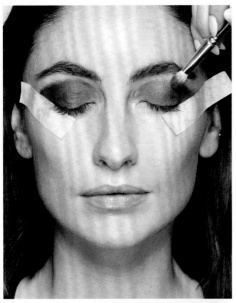

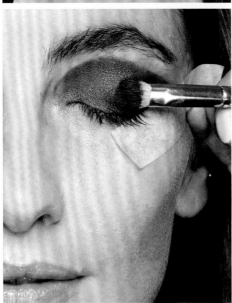

Step 1

Carefully attach a strip of masking tape to your cheek from the corner of your eye to the corner of your brow. If you're brows are slightly short, make sure you follow the brow-mapping section on pages 28–29 before you try this look. Using a blending brush, apply your darkest bronze shadow all over the lid, out to the tape and into the socket.

Step 2

Next, take your medium copper shadow and blend this over your eyelid with the same brush, avoiding the socket, as you want this to remain bronze.

Step 3

Gently remove the masking tape from your face – I like to do this with my head tilted forwards to shake off any excess shadow that may have fallen onto the tape or cheek. You'll see the gorgeous triangular shape that you've created.

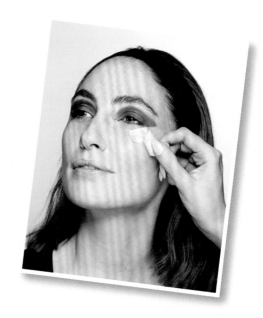

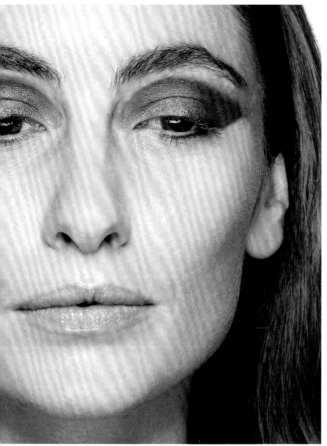

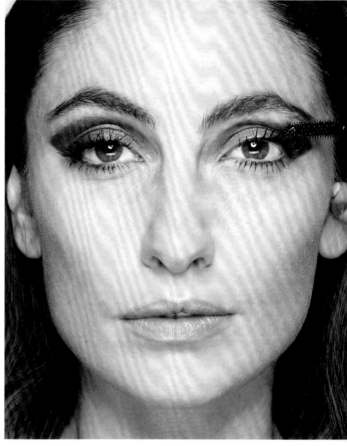

Step 4

Pat the lightest, slightly gold shadow into the centre of the lid using your ring finger and buff gently with a clean fluffy blending brush. Next, pat on a little bronze glitter for added shimmer.

Step 5

Finally, add two coats of black mascara and some false lashes (see pages 38–43) to go all-out glamour!

Colour removal
Use a cotton pad with a little make-up remover to remove any stray shadow before applying your base.

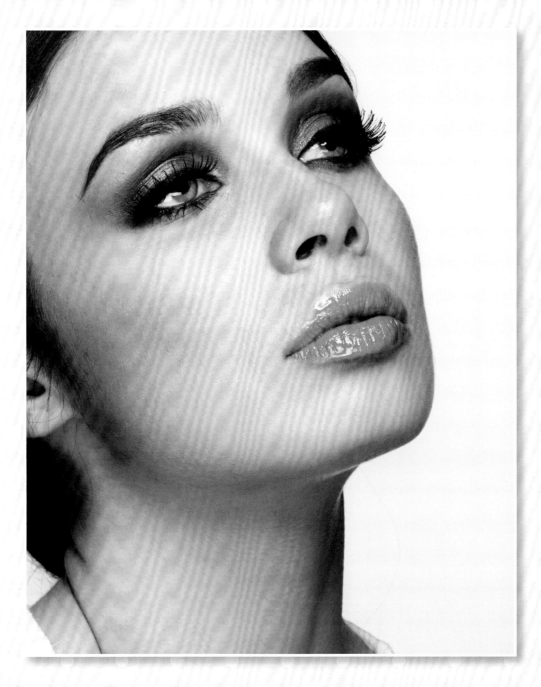

Apply a thicker line of liner to the top lash line before applying mascara for a really dramatic finish. A subtle use of highlighter under your brows will also give you an instant eye lift.

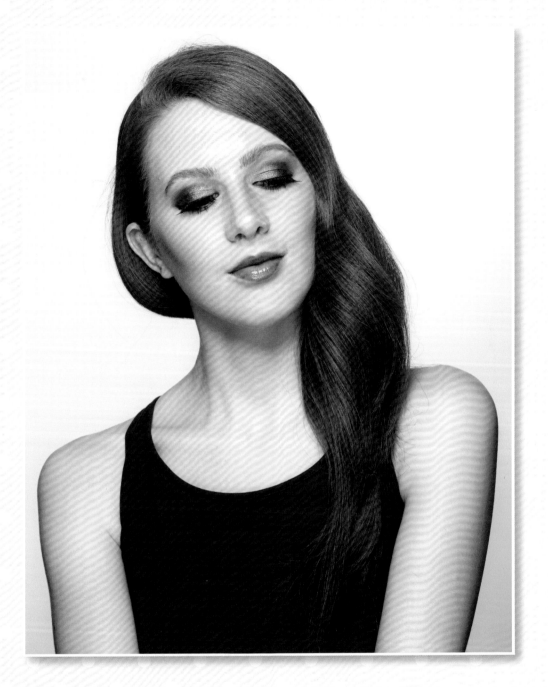

The copper tones of this bronze smoky eye look incredible with red hair.
Apply the lightest gold shade right into the inner corner to brighten the look.

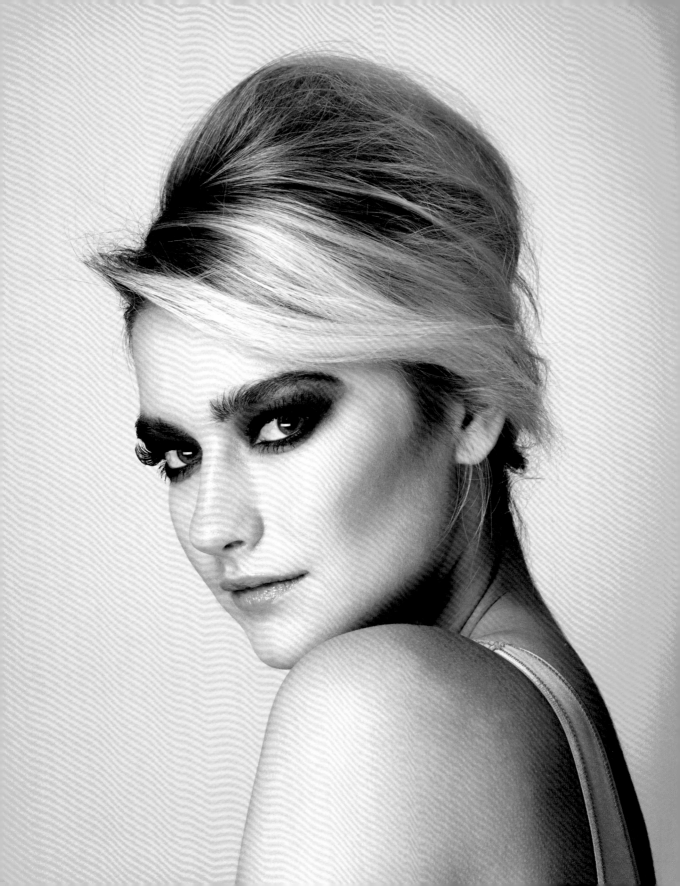

Colourful smoky eye in 30 minutes

Okay, ladies, are you ready to have some fun? That's what this look is all about! And trust me, in half an hour you're going to come out looking gorgeous. This is a three-tone look, so you want to pick colours that complement each other. I'm going for midnight blue, rich purple and hot pink. This look can look messy at first, but don't worry, it will all come together, and remember, with colourful eye shadow looks you'll do your base afterwards, so don't worry if the shadow drops under the eye.

All you need...

blending brush

hard-angled brush

pencil brush

cotton bud/swab

three colourful eye shadows (or a 3-colour eye-shadow palette)

black gel eye liner

black kohl eye liner

black mascara

1 pair strip lashes

eyelash glue

make-up remover

colourful eye shadows

strip lashes

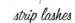

black kohl eye liner

black mascara

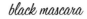

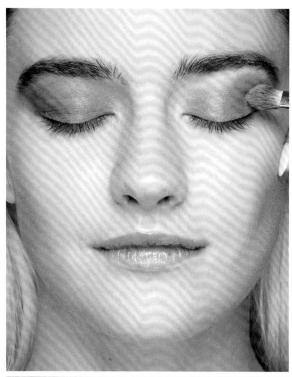

Wipe out!
Use a small strip of masking tape to quickly remove any pesky bits of eye shadow that fall on the cheeks.

Step 1

I start with the hot pink eye shadow (or the lightest shade). It's important that this shade literally looks like the most beautiful smoky clouds, so it's all about the blending! Apply the shadow all over the lid, into the socket and slightly above and out using a blending brush. Now, blend, blend, blend to build up the colour evenly for the super-smooth, airbrush finish you need. Next, apply the same colour under the lower lash line using a hard-angled brush. You are framing the eye with this bright shade. There should be no visible hard edges with this colour, so be patient and keep blending!

Step 2

Take the rich purple (or medium shade). Buff it onto the eyelid and into the socket of the eye using the same fluffy blending brush you used before. Buff it outwards slightly, but don't take it up as high as the pink shadow. Use a pencil brush to blend this shadow under the lash line as you did previously but again, not as low as you went with the pink.

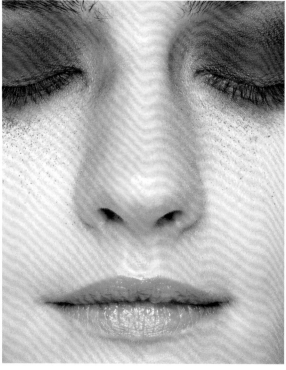

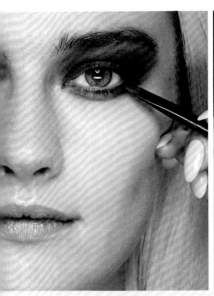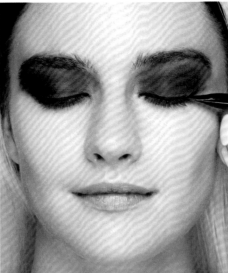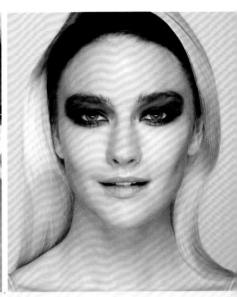

Step 3

Now, for the midnight blue eye shadow (or the darkest shade). This should be applied onto the lid section of the eye only. Blend it backwards and forwards with your blending brush but don't take it any higher than the socket of the eye. Next, use a damp hard-angled brush and apply the midnight blue shadow directly under the lower lash line to add depth.

Step 4

It's time to line! Apply a jet-black gel eye liner to the top lash line. End the liner where your eye ends. Then, using the same liner, draw a third of the way under the lower lash line, hugging the lashes as closely as you can. Blend the liner gently with a cotton bud/swab to soften it, then apply a black kohl liner to the waterline. Turn to pages 98–101 to see exactly how to do this.

Step 5

Apply two layers of black mascara, bottom lashes first (see pages 36–37). Finish with a strip of false lashes, following the instructions on pages 38–41.

Now for the clean-up. Remove any eye shadow that's dropped onto the cheeks with make-up remover using a cotton pad before perfecting your base and lips. Get your hair did, slip on a pair of your favourite shoes and get out on the town!

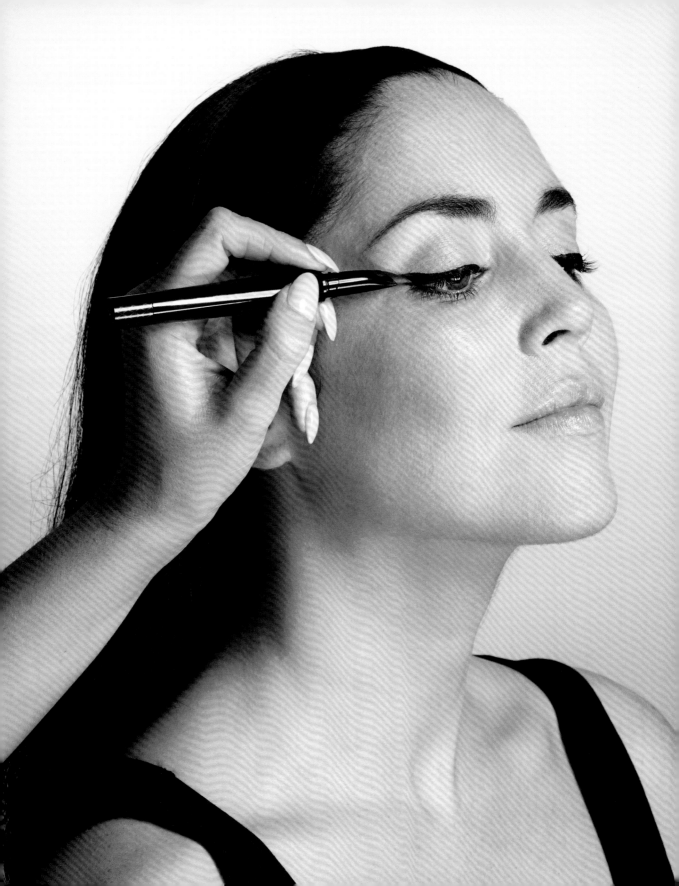

Liner looks

Eye liner is like riding a bike: when you've got it, you've got it! It does take a bit of practice but it should never take longer than 15 minutes unless you're going for something really graphic. Pick and choose from this selection of quick liner looks to find the perfect look for you. Remember, you can wear any of these looks by themselves, or with any other eye look in this book.

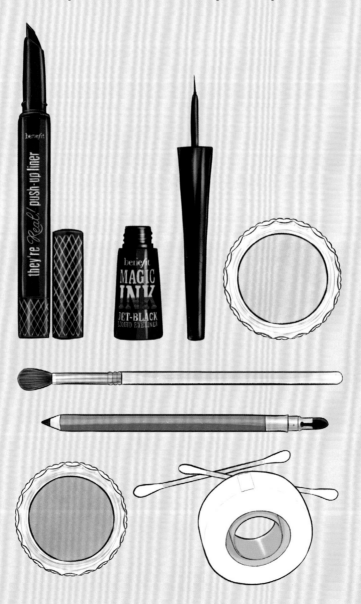

Fine and defined in 5 minutes

Sometimes we just want something fine and defined, like a good glass of wine or a pair of Louboutin Pigalle shoes. But this is a book about eye looks, so I'd better stick to the point! Liner will give you bigger, more beautiful eyes in seconds, whatever your age. A fine liner look is quick, easy and effective. You can wear it on its own, or over eye shadow.

This look is great for everyday wear but also finishes off some of the more complicated smokin' eye looks on pages 46–87. And what's even better is that you only need two things to look this fabulous!

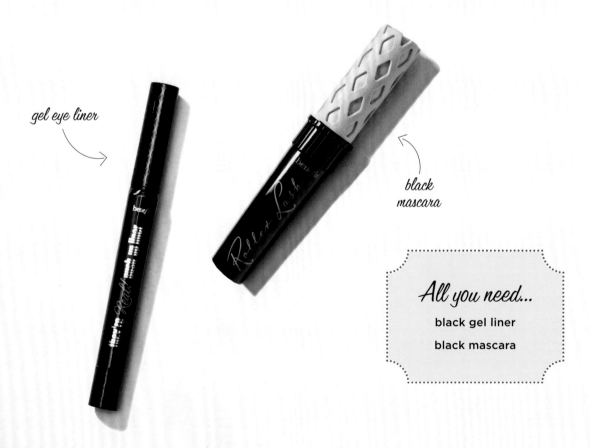

gel eye liner

black mascara

All you need...
black gel liner
black mascara

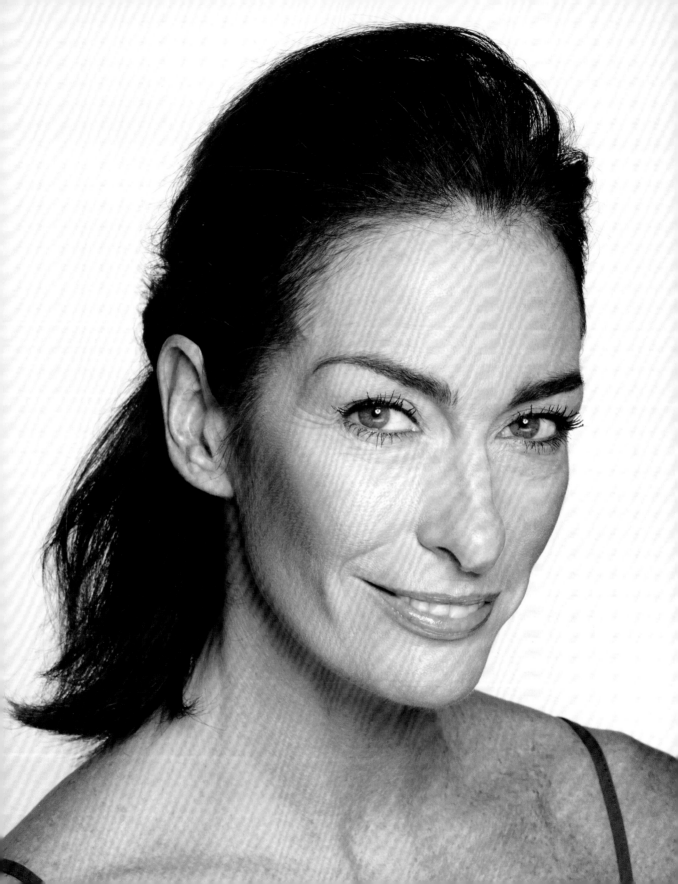

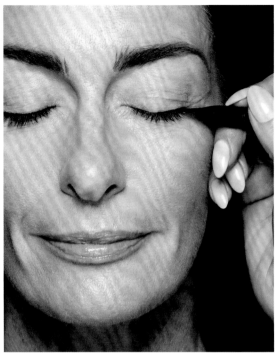

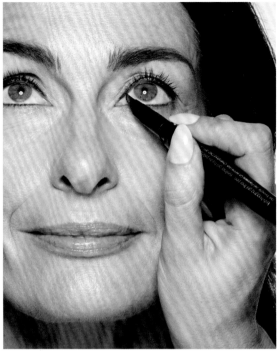

Step 1

Rest the liner on your top lashes – this will make sure you hug the lashes: there's nothing worse than a gappy eye look! Start in the centre of the eyelid and glide the liner to the outer corner of the eye. Be sure to stop where your lashes stop. If you take the line too far, it can make your eyes look droopy.

Step 2

Now glide the line to the inner corner of your eye. When you get really good, you'll be able to do a full line in one go, but even I still find this a quicker and neater way to do things.

Step 3

Add mascara to the bottom then top lashes (see pages 36–37) and you're done. So fine, so defined!

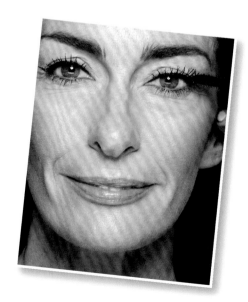

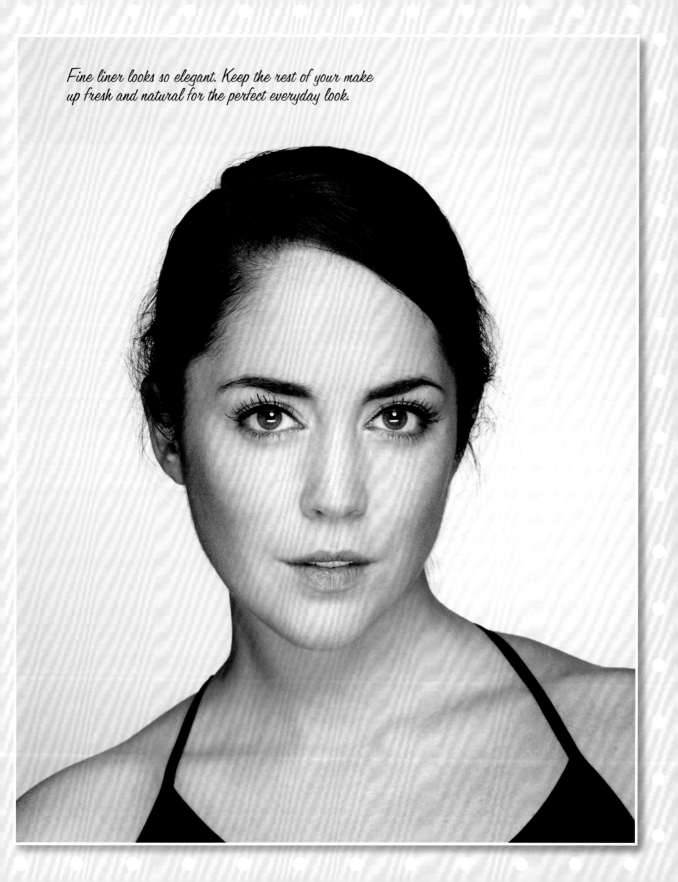

Fine liner looks so elegant. Keep the rest of your make up fresh and natural for the perfect everyday look.

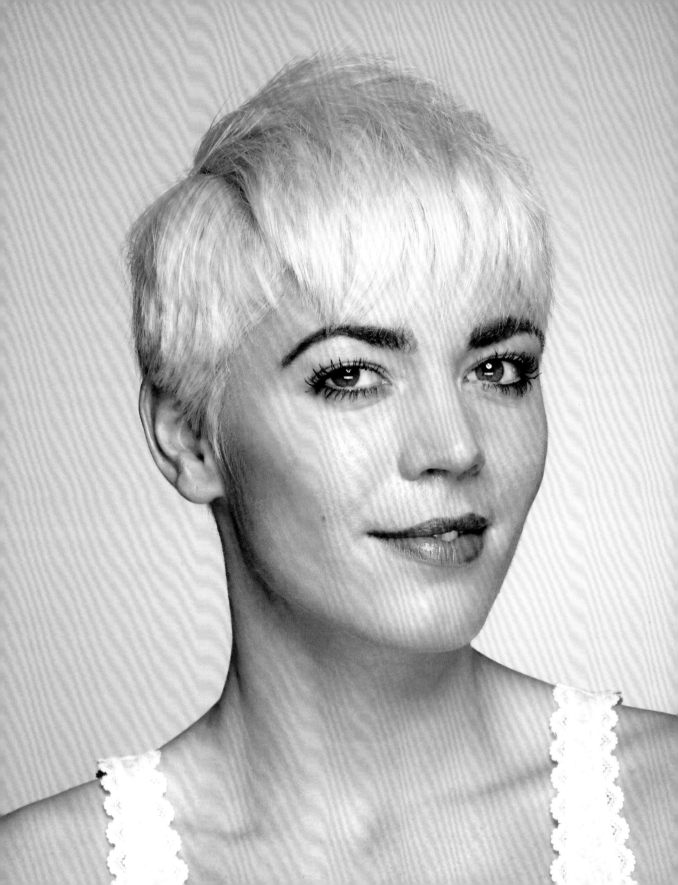

The under smoke in 5 minutes

Lining under the lower lash line can look really cool, but it's not for everyone. Give it a go, see what you think, but don't just assume that this look is for you. If it works for you, then don't be afraid to use any colour that you like.

You can also experiment with applying shadow in dots beneath the lower lash line for an edgier version of this rock 'n' roll look.

All you need...

pencil brush

cotton bud/swab

coloured eye shadow

black gel or liquid eye liner

blue mascara

black mascara

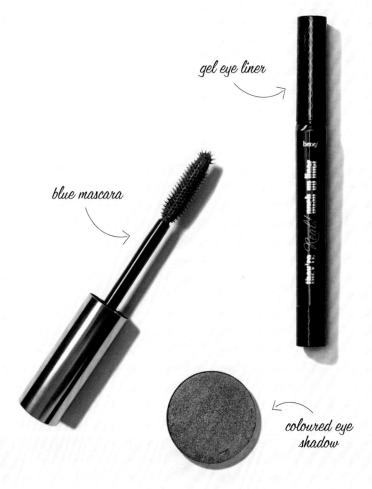

gel eye liner

blue mascara

coloured eye shadow

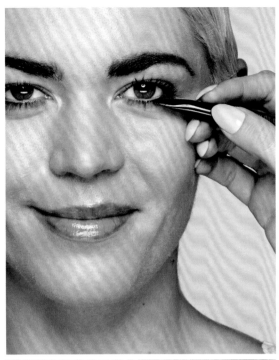

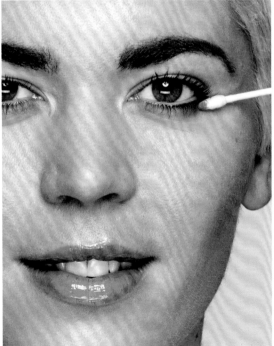

Step 1

Blend a thick line of eye shadow under the bottom lashes using a pencil brush. Then draw a fine line of black eye liner under the lower lash line – don't worry if it's not perfect because we're about to smudge!

Step 2

Take a cotton bud/swab and blend the liner and shadow underneath the bottom lashes to lightly smudge the line for a cool finish.

Step 3

Apply mascara (see pages 36–37) – I love to use blue mascara on the bottom lashes and black mascara on the top with this look. Blue mascara contrasts the beautifully coloured eye shadow you've built up beneath the bottom lashes, while black on top opens the eye for a bright but edgy look.

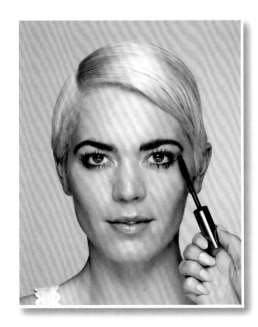

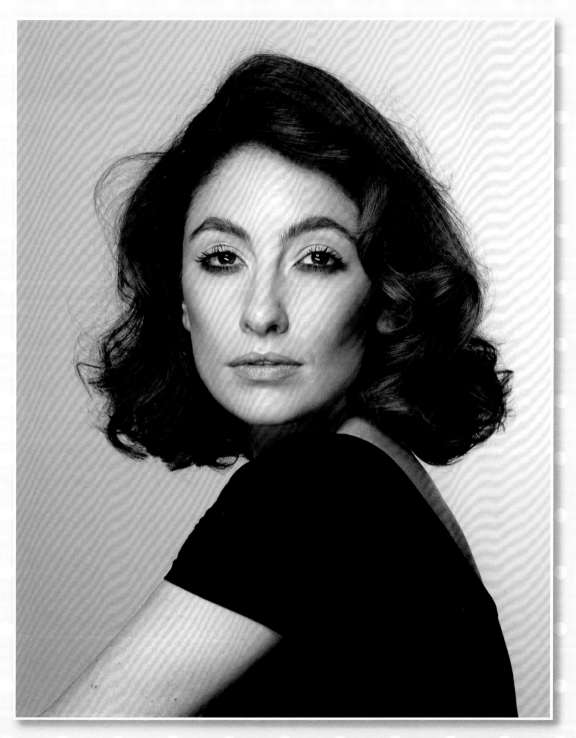

This look is perfect for experimenting with colour as it's super easy and you can use any eye shadow or liner that you like. Consult the colour chart on page 34 for tips on which colours to try first.

The waterline in 5 minutes

Throughout this book, I refer to applying liner to your waterline. This can really complete a look and is super-easy to do. It can feel a bit weird at first – I mean, you are sticking a pencil in your eye – so proceed carefully until you get the hang of it, because it's totally worth it!

Kohl eye liners are best for this look as they don't spread or smudge as quickly as shadows, gel or liquid eye liners could.

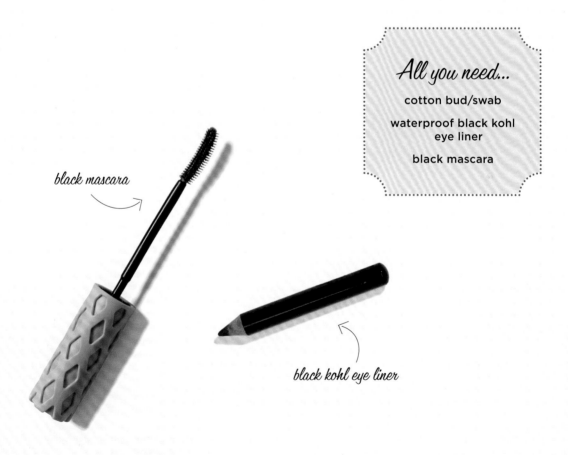

black mascara

black kohl eye liner

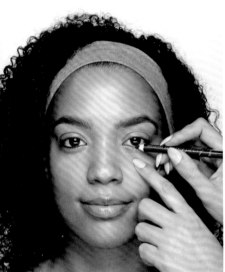

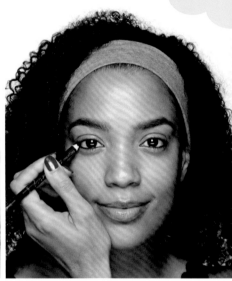

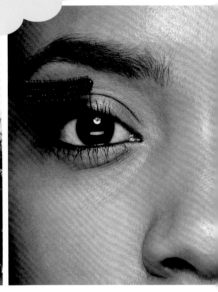

Back to black

Black eye liner defines and frames the eyes so is really versatile for all kinds of eye looks.

Step 1

Take a waterproof kohl pencil (make sure it's sharp). Gently pull under your lower lid to reveal the pink skin of the bottom waterline. Look straight into the mirror and apply the liner from one end to the other. Have a cotton bud on hand to dab away any tears from watery eyes. Repeat until you have the depth of colour your desire.

Step 2

Liner doesn't have to be bold and beautiful; it can also be used to create an illusion. If you have sparse, fine lashes, then lining your top

waterline could change your whole look! Look down and gently pull your top lashes outwards to reveal the pink skin of the top waterline. Draw a line on the top waterline as you would the bottom and go over it two or three times for depth of colour.

As a make-up artist, I always ask my client if they would prefer to line their top waterline themselves, as this area can be super-sensitive.

Step 3

Apply mascara (see pages 36–37). Voilà! Thicker-looking lashes in seconds!

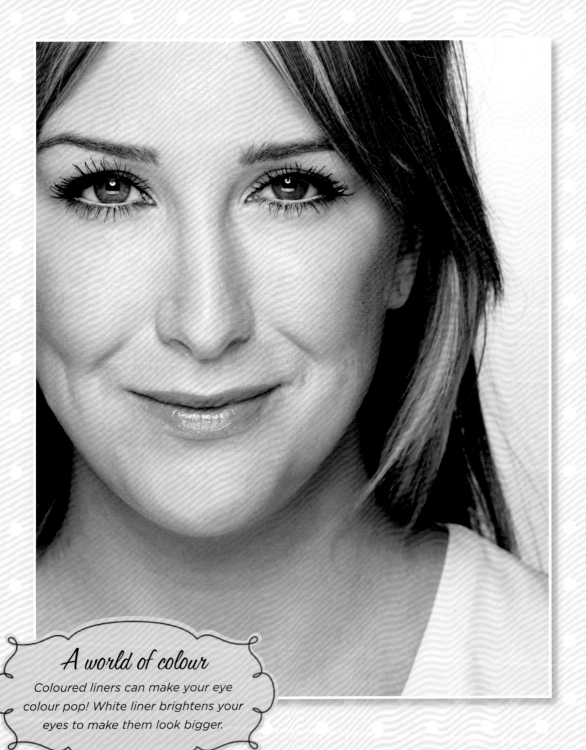

A world of colour

Coloured liners can make your eye colour pop! White liner brightens your eyes to make them look bigger.

Behind the scenes at London Fashion Week

Twice a year I have the honour of diving into the craziness that is London Fashion Week. I've worked with the wonderful Matthew Williamson for six seasons now. We share a love for colour, anything that sparkles and flamingos!

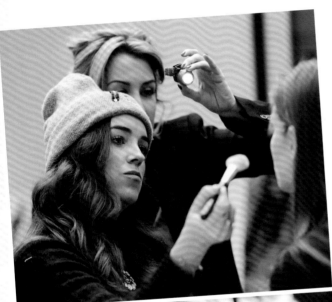

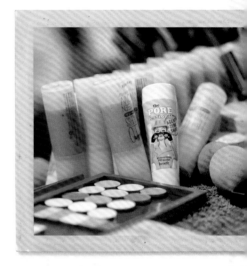

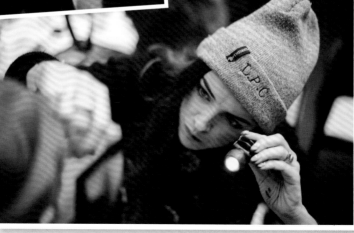

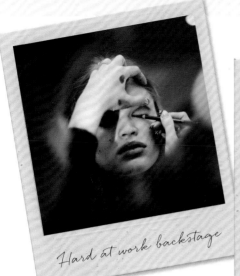

Hard at work backstage

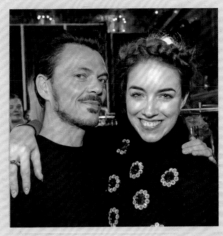

Me and Matthew

I wanted to give you a taster of what it's like behind the scenes at one of the biggest shows of the season.

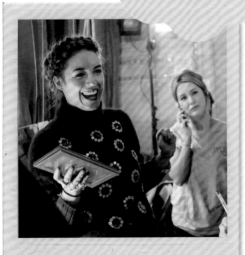

Me and my assistant Lauren

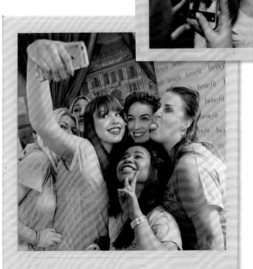

There's always time for a selfie

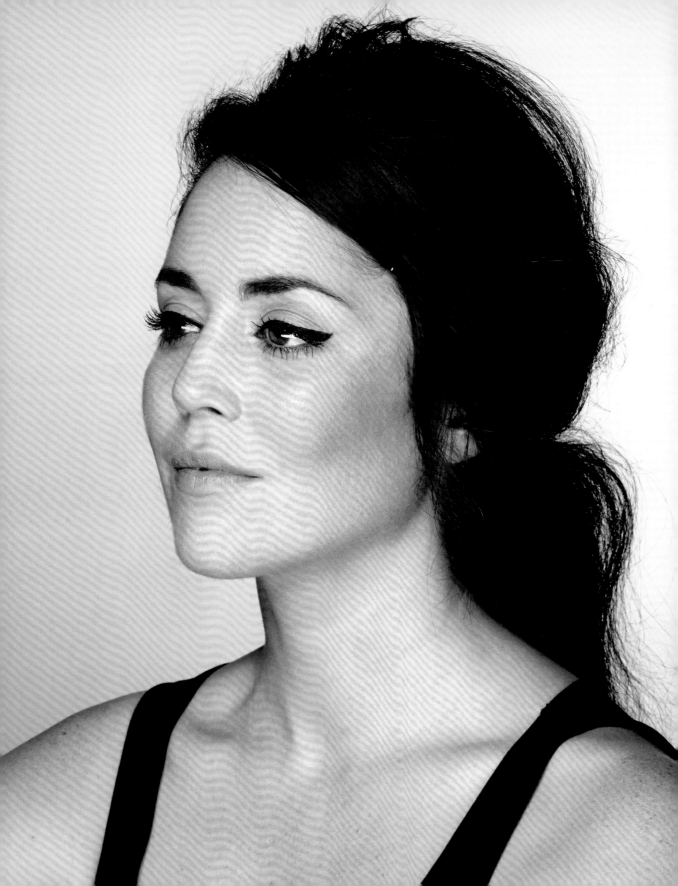

The classic flick in 15 minutes

Every day I get asked how to create the perfect classic flick! It's such an iconic look, made famous by the likes of Marilyn Monroe and Audrey Hepburn. However, it's also one of the biggest beauty dilemmas out there, as it always seems so complicated. I've allowed 15 minutes for this look, but the more you practise, the quicker you will get. You'll be classic flick experts in no time, as this look is easier than you think, girls – just follow these simple steps.

Pick the colour and type of liner that you would like to use. Black is classic, and I prefer gel liner because it gives a matte finish, but that doesn't mean you can't use one of the many coloured liners out there.

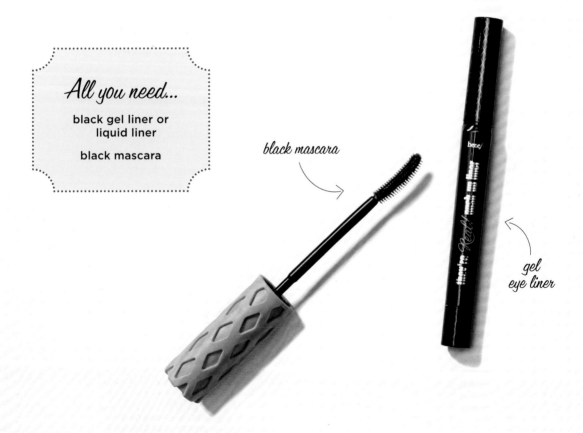

All you need...

black gel liner or liquid liner

black mascara

black mascara

gel eye liner

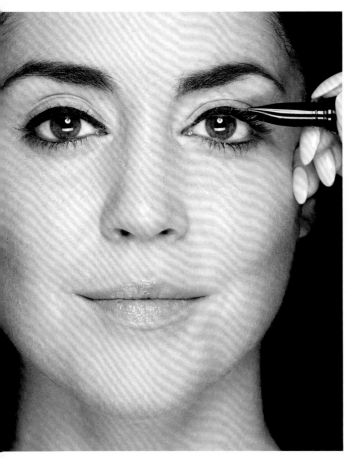

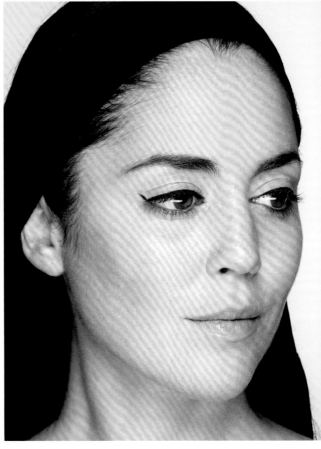

Step 1

I always start by applying my liner in the centre of the upper eyelid – I just find it easier to see what I'm doing that way. So, starting in the centre, draw a line each way along the top lash line, as close to the lashes as possible.

Step 2

From the outside corner of your eye, draw a line angled upwards, approximately 5 mm/ ⅛ inch in length, towards the end of your brow.

Join the dots

Don't feel like you have to draw the line in one go. You can always draw small lines and then join the dots.

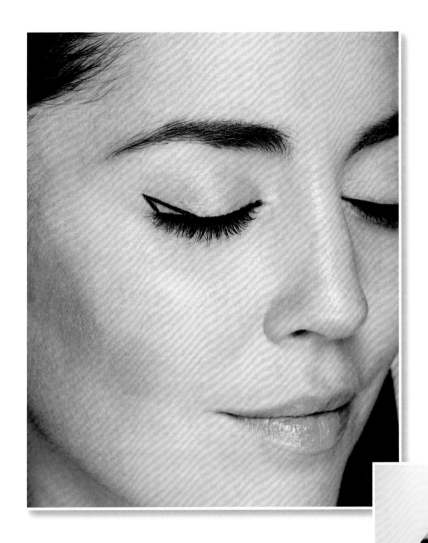

Step 3

From the tip of this line, draw back towards the lash line about a third of the way along the eye.

Step 4

Fill in the gap and apply mascara (see pages 36–37). And that is how to get a classic flick in less than 15 minutes!

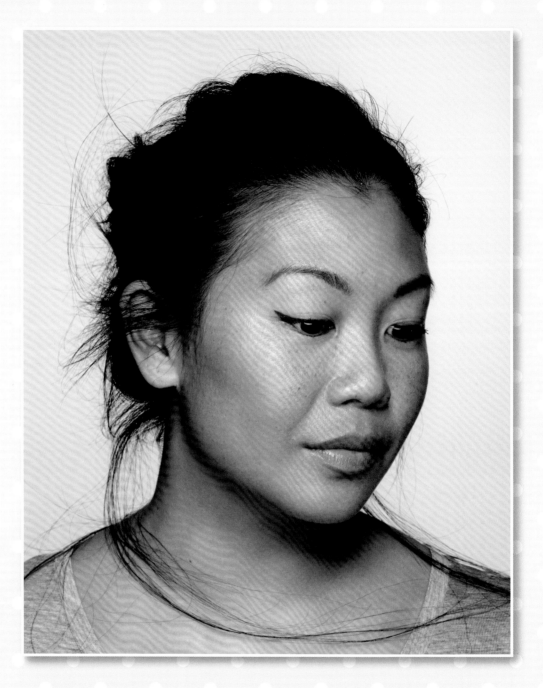

A classic flick on Asian eyes lifts and opens the eye beautifully. For more tips and tricks for different eye shapes, see page 35. Coloured eyeliners are so fun. Once you've got the hang of the flick, give it a go in any colour you like.

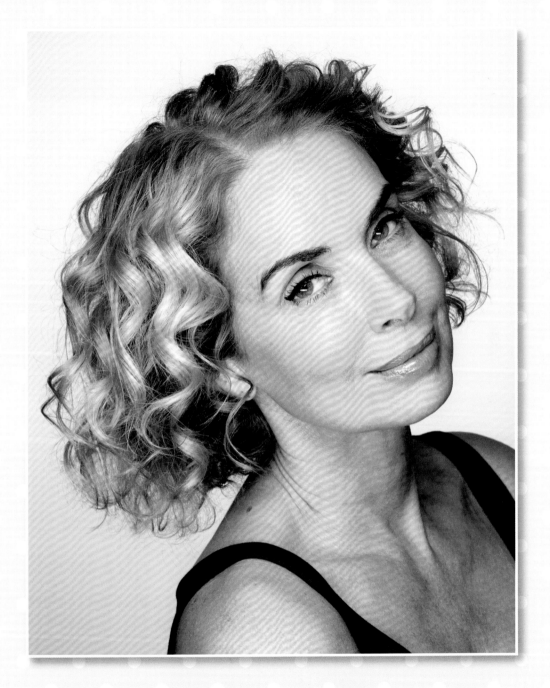

Don't be afraid to try a classic flick if you are more mature. It can look fantastic. However, if you have hooded eyes (see eye shapes on page 35), stick to the Fine and defined look on pages 90-93.

Graphic liner in 5 minutes

Graphic liner can be so cool and so quick. If you've only got 5 minutes and you want to stand out from the crowd, forget the rules and follow these simple steps.

Pick your eye shadow – yes, we're using an eye shadow instead of a liner here – but rest assured, we'll be drawing a line with it! Colourwise, any colour works for this, but the brighter the better, in my opinion. Keep the rest of the face quite plain: hair pinned, nude cheeks and brushed up brows, so that your eyes do all the talking.

All you need...

pointed cotton bud/swab

pink eye shadow

Vaseline jelly

black mascara
(optional)

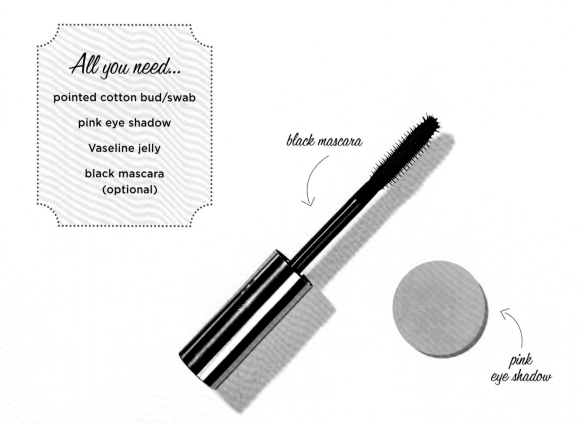

black mascara

pink
eye shadow

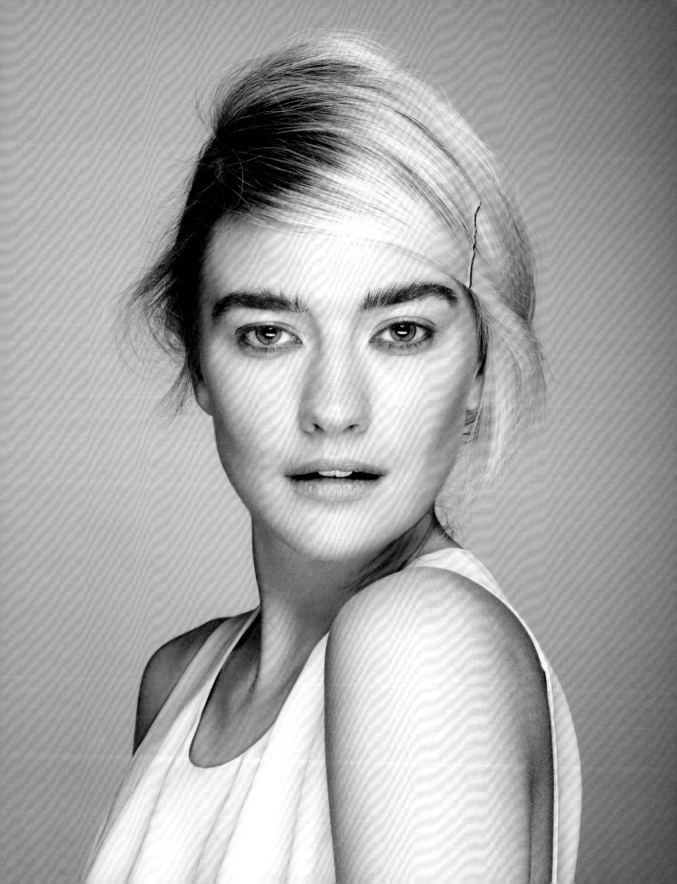

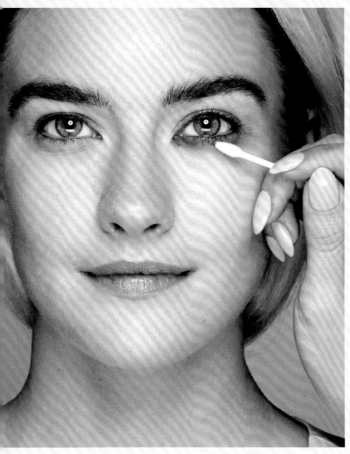

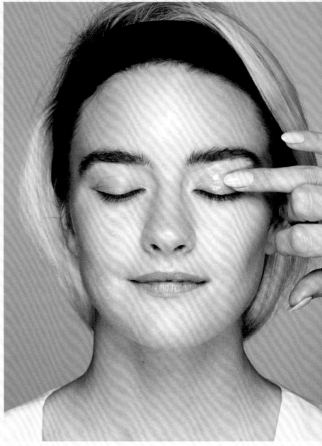

Step 1

No brushes necessary! Pick up a cotton bud/swab (the ones with the pointy ends are best for this), dip it in your shadow and draw a line under the lower lash line that starts from the inner corner of your eye, and ends halfway along. Blend slightly.

Step 2

Add mascara if you like, but personally, for this look, I prefer no mascara and just a touch of Vaseline jelly carefully patted onto the upper eyelid using your ring finger.

Who knew graphic liner could be so simple, hey? And who knew you didn't need a liner at all?

See-through sheen

Apply a thin layer of Vaseline jelly all over the eyelid, right up to the brow for a shine that won't quit.

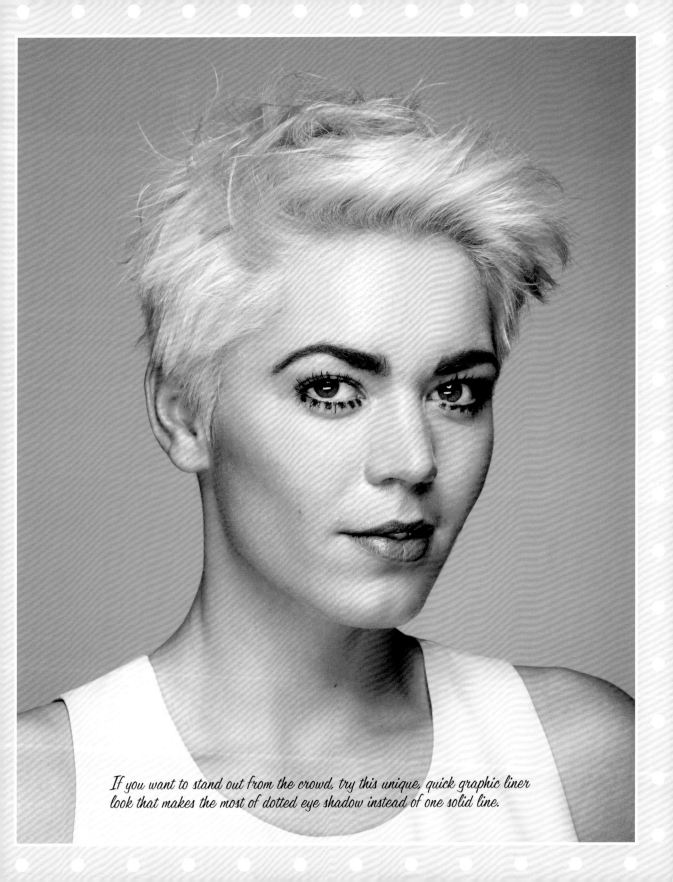

If you want to stand out from the crowd, try this unique, quick graphic liner look that makes the most of dotted eye shadow instead of one solid line.

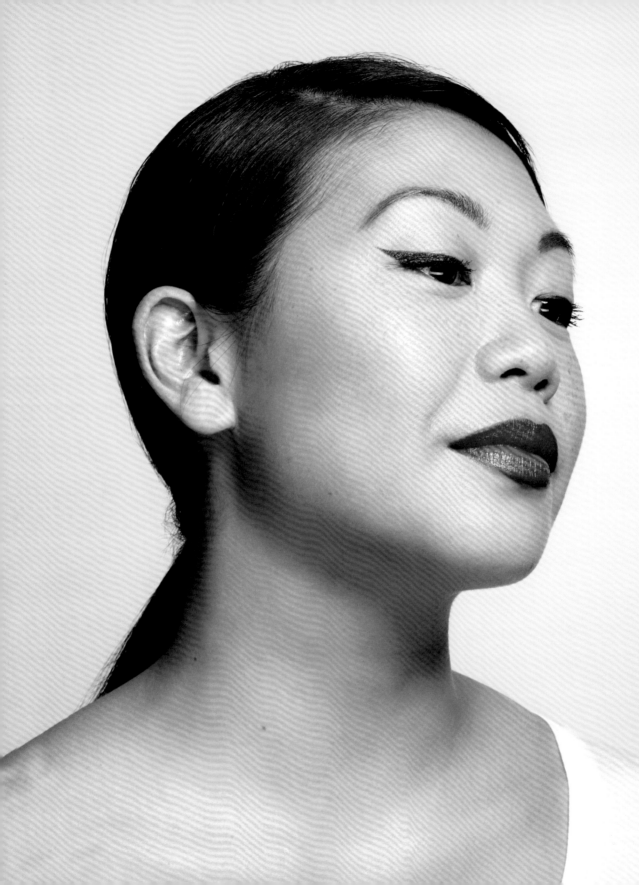

The big flick in 15 minutes

This is one of my faves! If I want drama, then this is my go-to look. Large liner is super-cool, and really flattering on the eye, too.

Pick the colour and type of liner you would like to use. Gel or liquid liner works best here. Liner aside, you only really need a lick of black mascara, but I love a striking bright lip colour for added drama with this Hollywood look.

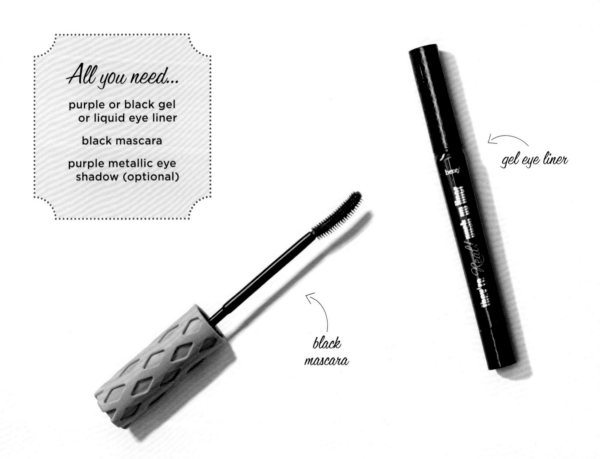

All you need...

purple or black gel or liquid eye liner

black mascara

purple metallic eye shadow (optional)

gel eye liner

black mascara

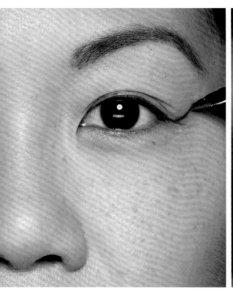 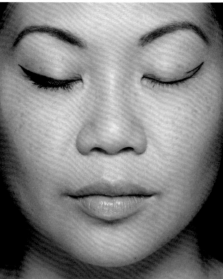 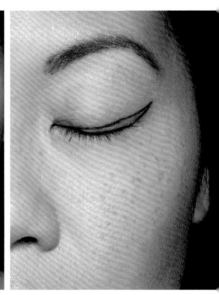

Step 1

Unlike the classic flick, for this look we're going to start with the wing. Draw a line from the corner of your eye, angled upwards towards the end of your brow. The longer this line, the more dramatic the look, so go as far as you dare.

Step 2

From the tip of this line, draw back towards the centre of the eye, but stop as you reach the middle of the eye.

Step 3

Continue the line down towards the inner corner of the eye.

Step 4

Fill in the gaps of the shape you have created. Add lashings of mascara (see pages 36–37). The big flick is back!

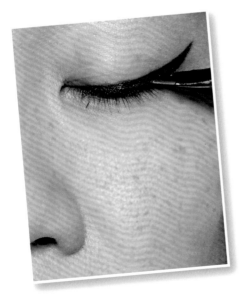

Line up, line up!

Be brave and give this look a go with any colour liner – the bigger and brighter the better!

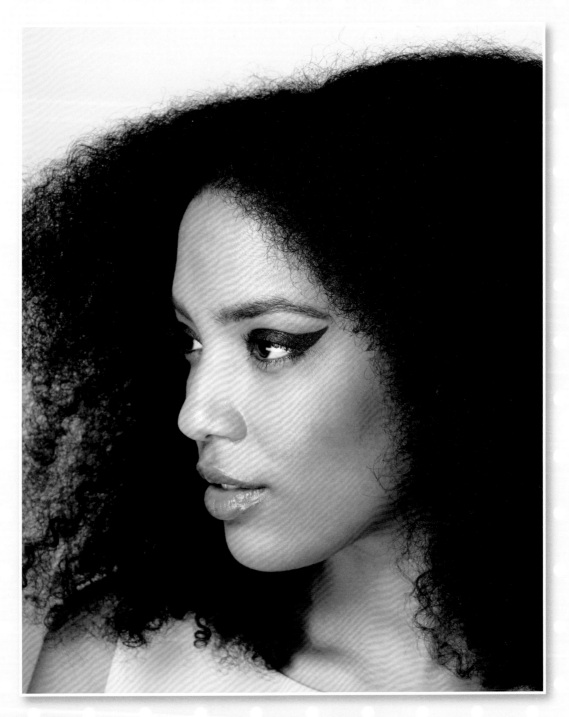

For a more textured finish, carefully go over the liner with a similar-coloured metallic eyeshadow using a hard-angled brush.

Graphic liner in 30 minutes

I heart this graduated liner look. First create a simple shape around the eyelid using gel or liquid eye liner then colour in the corners using a kohl pencil. It's super-cool, but does take a bit of practice.

Start by mastering the Fine and defined liner look on pages 90–93, as it forms the basis of this look, then go graphic!

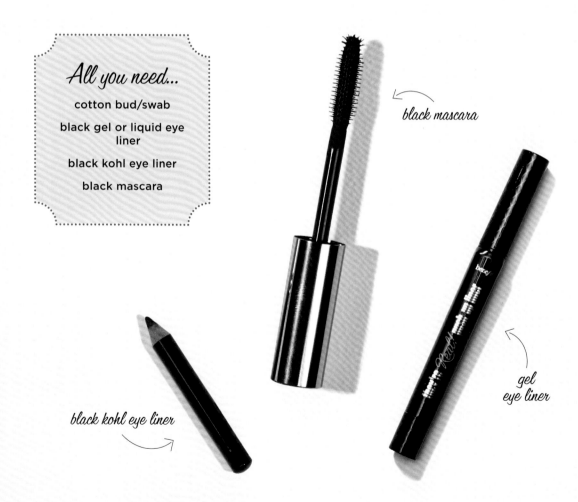

All you need...
cotton bud/swab

black gel or liquid eye liner

black kohl eye liner

black mascara

black mascara

gel eye liner

black kohl eye liner

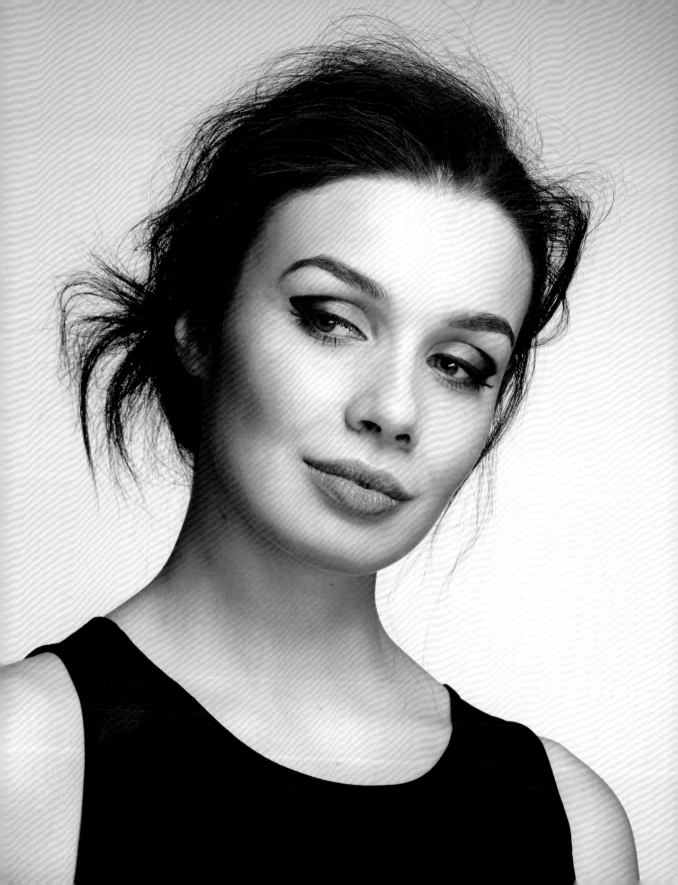

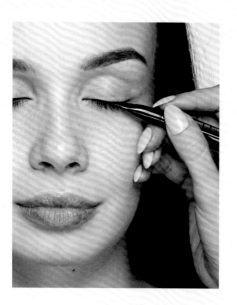

Step 1

Draw a thin line along the top lash line using either a gel or a liquid eyeliner. I prefer a gel, as I love a matte finish. Get this as close to the lash line as possible.

Mind the gap

Fill in any little gaps that appear along your lash line using a kohl pencil for fuller-looking lashes in an instant.

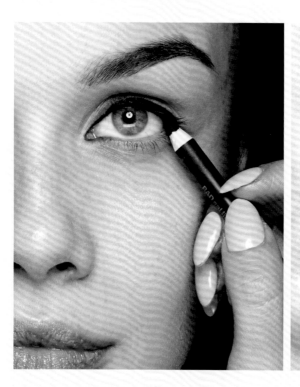

Step 2

Carefully apply black kohl pencil in the top waterline (see pages 98–101) for a really polished final look.

Step 3

Draw a line straight up from the corner of the eye towards the socket as you would for a classic or big flick.

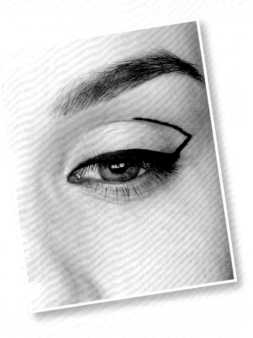

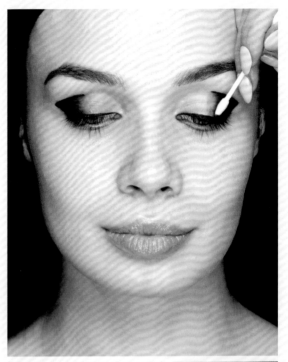

Step 4

Draw a line following the socket of the eye, moving towards the centre. Stop halfway along the socket.

Step 5

Take a black kohl pencil and shade in the shape you have created, stopping halfway into the shape. Use a cotton bud/swab to blend the pencil towards the centre of the eye. This gives a gorgeous smoky effect without needing to use any eye shadow.

Step 6

Add two layers of mascara (see pages 36–37). Trust me, all your friends will be wanting you to recreate this beaut of a look on them!

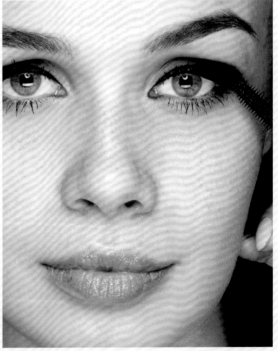

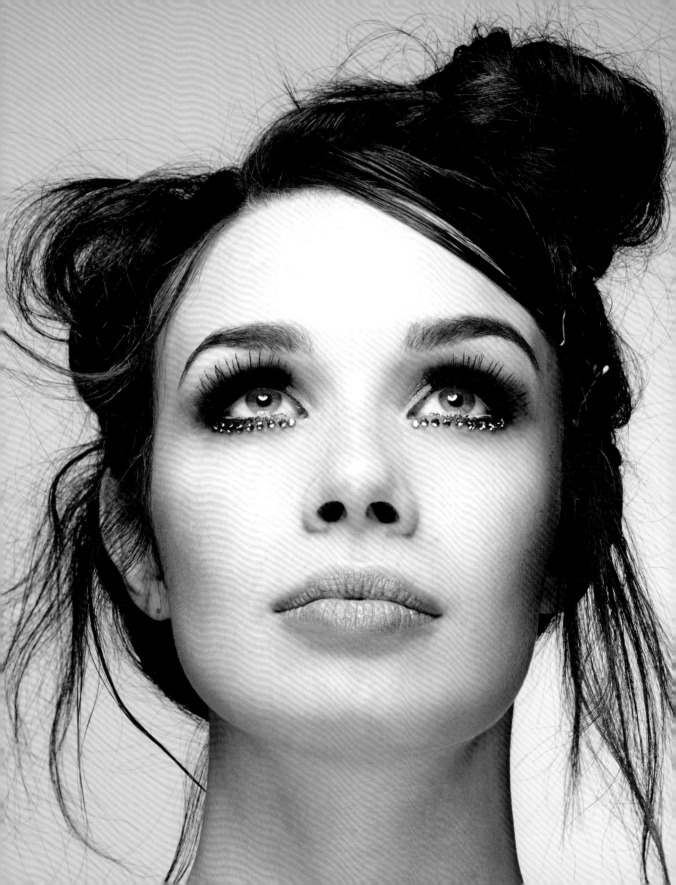

Now to wow!

Okay, so I'm assuming you can now do a smoky eye with your eyes closed and a classic flick while on a moving train, standing up, during rush hour! For my final looks I thought I'd go super-creative and show you how to create a few looks that I have purpose-made for either the catwalk or a magazine shoot. These looks are unique and beautiful, so give them a go and have fun!

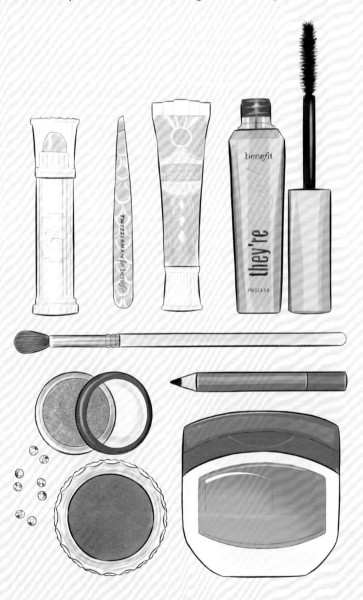

All that glitters in 30 minutes

If you ask my friends what runs through my veins, they'd all say glitter!
I love glitter!!! I put it on cakes, on cards, on my clothes and I especially *love* a glittery eye!

Top tip: always do your eye make-up first when using glitter. It tends to end up everywhere and you don't want to ruin your base. Have some masking tape to hand (I always have a roll in my kit) as it's the best thing to remove glitter from the face, and it doesn't stick to the skin like normal sellotape. Now you're ready for some shimmer and shine!

Pick your colours. I suggest one cream or powder shadow as the base and a glitter that's of a similar shade to complement it. Of course, you can also go for any colour glitter you like.

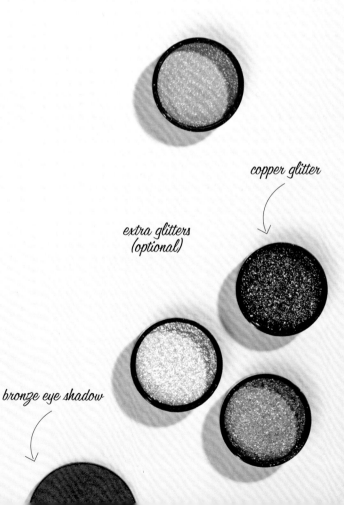

All you need...

blending brushes

tissue/Kleenex

pencil brush

eye shadow

glitter

Vaseline jelly (optional)

waterproof black kohl eye liner

black mascara

copper glitter

extra glitters
(optional)

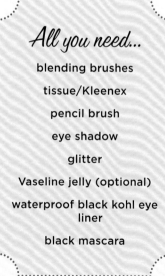

bronze eye shadow

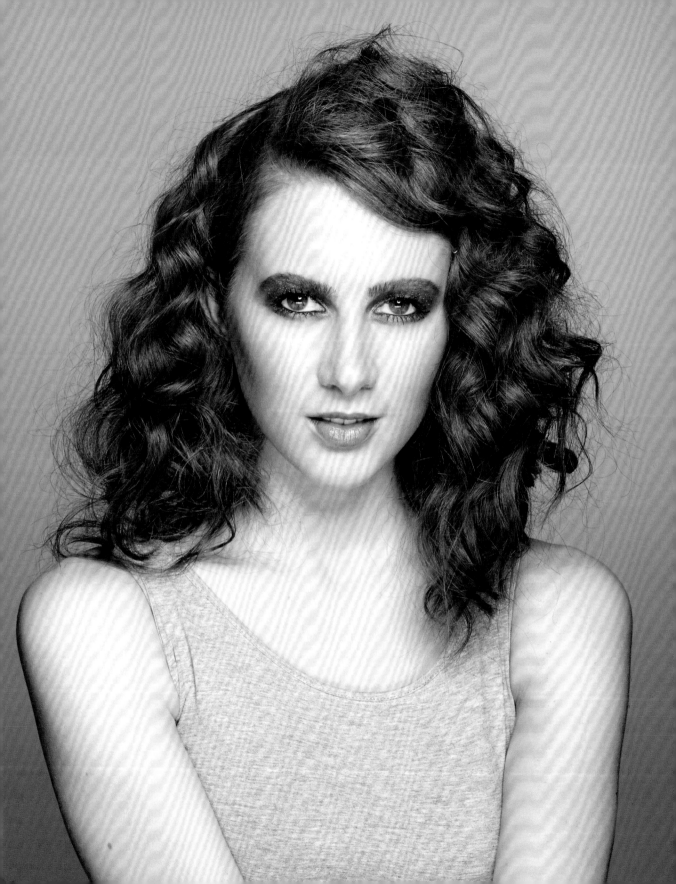

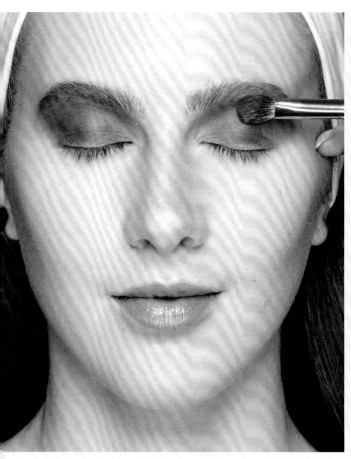
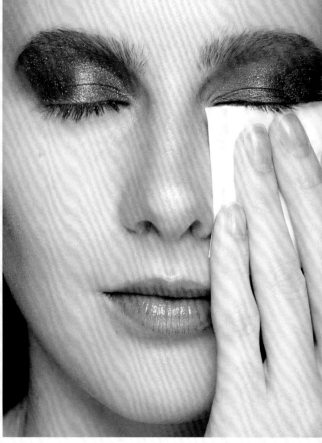

Step 1

Buff your base colour over the lid and into the socket using a fluffy blending brush. I've taken the shadow all the way up to the brows for a '70s disco vibe with this look, which gives you loads of room to add glitter, next. Spend a good amount of time blending and building up this colour to make sure there are no hard edges.

Step 2

Time for the GLITTER! I've chosen a bronze shade to complement the shadow. If you can, hold a tissue/Kleenex under your eye to catch any of the glitter that falls – trust me, it will! Use a flat eye-shadow brush to apply the glitter all over the lid. Pat it in place with your ring finger for a gentle touch and layer it up until you are satisfied that you are shimmery enough.

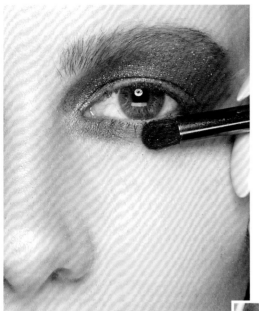

Stuck on you
Apply a small amount of Vaseline jelly over the base colour before you apply the glitter to help it stick.

Step 3
Blend the eye shadow you used for your base under the lower lash line using a pencil brush to frame the eye.

Step 4
To finish the look, apply black liner on the top and bottom waterline (see pages 98–101). Then, of course, add tonnes of black mascara. Shimmer and shine, now it's definitely party time!

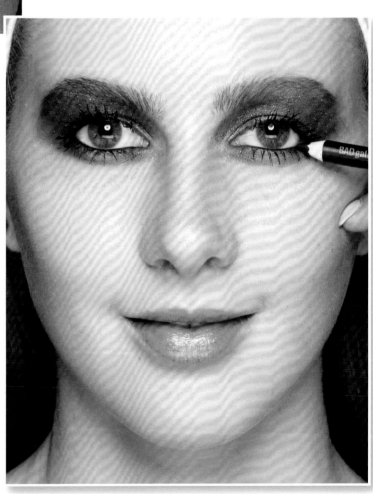

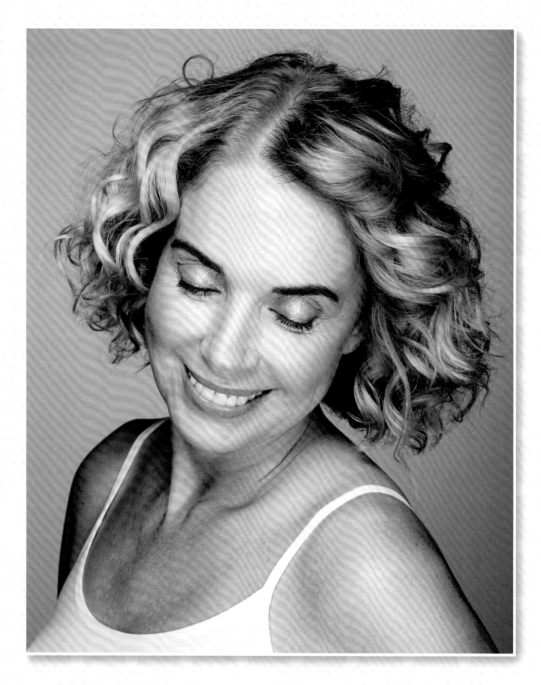

A wash of glitter on more mature eyes looks fantastic over a primed eyelid.
Stick to golds and silvers for a natural finish.

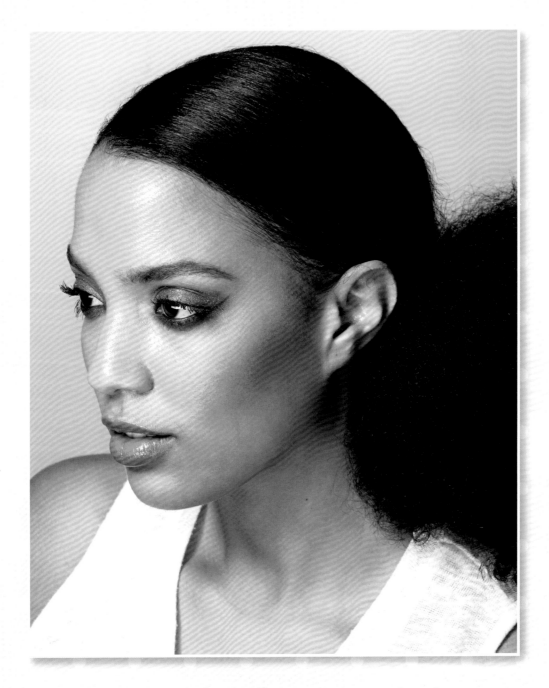

Try adding glitter over a smoky eye. Match the glitter to the colour of your eye shadow and head to the dancefloor immediately!

Get the gloss in 15 minutes

You can add a bit of clear lip gloss or Vaseline jelly over any of the smoky eye looks in this book. Just be aware that it does move the eye shadow. This can look really cool, but it can also look really messy if you want your make-up to last for 12 hours or more! However, it's perfect for a night out if you're in the mood for something a bit different.

This technique looks amazing with metallic cream shadows. It also looks great applied over lipstick! That's right, I'm going to use a lipstick on the eye. Anything creamy is fab, as it sits better underneath the gloss than eye shadow.

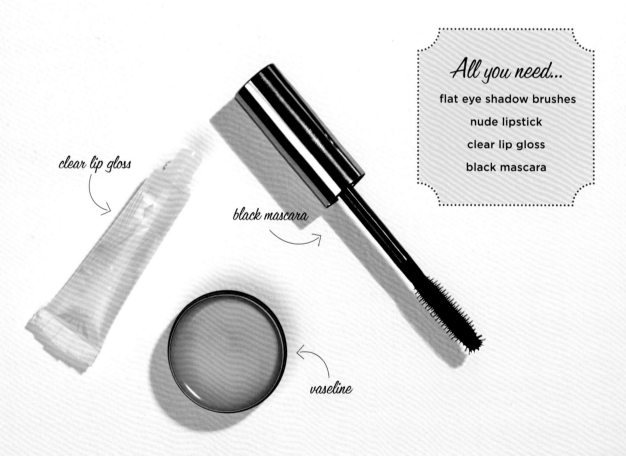

clear lip gloss

black mascara

vaseline

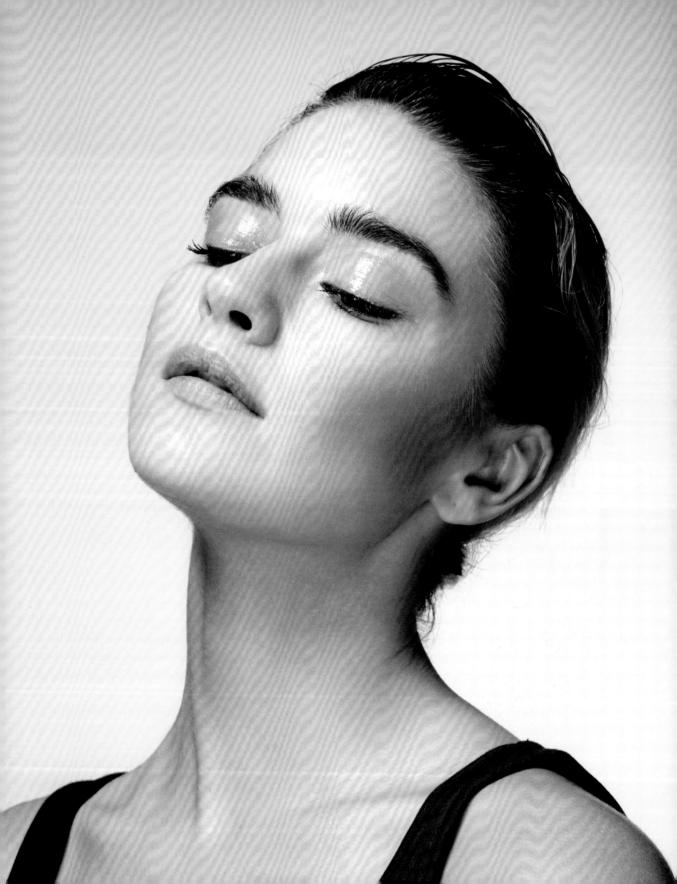

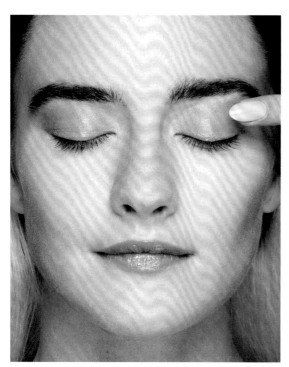

Bare all

Use the same shade of nude lipstick on eyes and lips for real bare-faced chic.

Step 1

Layer on your colour. As I'm using a lipstick, I'm going to use a flat shadow brush to layer it up. I'm then going to blend with my fingers instead of a brush, as the warmth of the fingertips will help to manipulate the lipstick.

Step 2

Add a few layers of mascara (see pages 36–37). Make sure it's perfectly dry before you add the gloss.

Step 3

Using a clean, flat eye shadow brush, apply your chosen gloss over the top of the eye colour. Don't buff it in, pat it on carefully. You want it to be smooth, glossy and glorious!

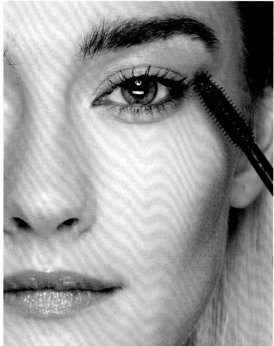

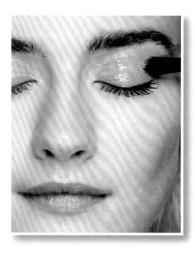

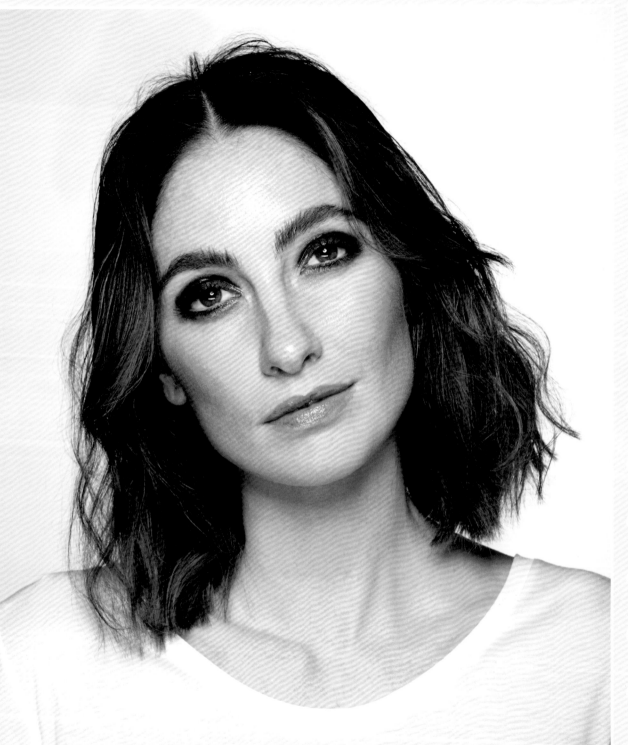

*Make a smoky eye glossy by patting a gloss over a Classic smoky eye
(see pages 48-51, 62-65 and 74-77) to add a real edge to your look.*

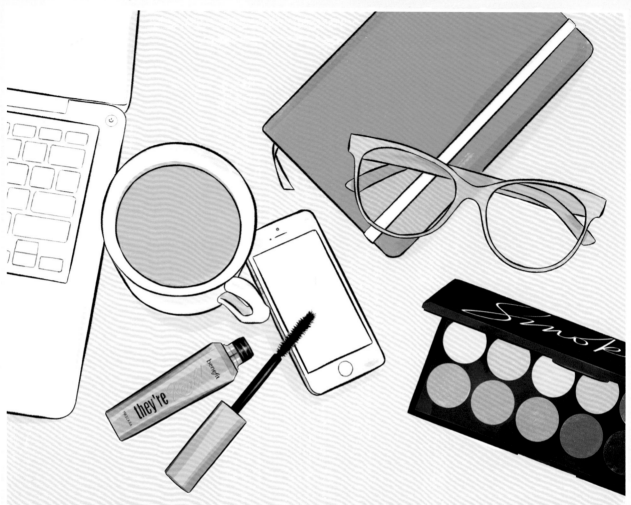

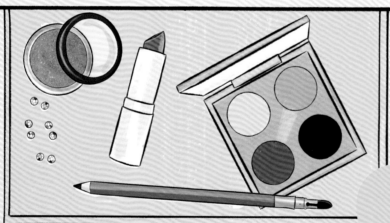

Disco nap

White and pale pink
eye shadow brightens
tired eyes.

I've had many occasions where I've got halfway through the day, then emailed a few girlfriends and organized a last-minute night out! And, why not, hey? The spontaneous nights are usually the best, right? Getting yourself glam with little to no notice may seem impossible if you don't have the right products with you and that is why I'm going to tell you which six products to keep in your desk drawer to literally take you from desk to dancefloor.

From desk to dancefloor

Bright lipstick

Nothing changes your look more than a gorgeous bright lipstick.
I love using a lip stain followed by a lipstick for a cocktail-proof pout.
Remember, you can also use lipstick as a blusher.

Eye-shadow palette

These are great to keep in your desk drawer. Taking your eye make-up from a natural nude to a classic smoke adds instant impact.

Moisturizer

This is one of my top tips! To freshen up your base, rub a small amount of moisturizer between your hands and then lightly pat over your face. This will give you an instant dewy glow without taking off your make-up or needing to apply it again!

Glitter

Nothing says party more than a touch of glitter. Patting glitter into the centre of your eye will transport you to the dancefloor instantly!

False lashes

I'm hoping you're now a false lash pro, so applying these at 5:30 pm will be easy! Luscious lashes really add that wow factor.

This book!

I mean, you've got to remember how to do the looks, right?!

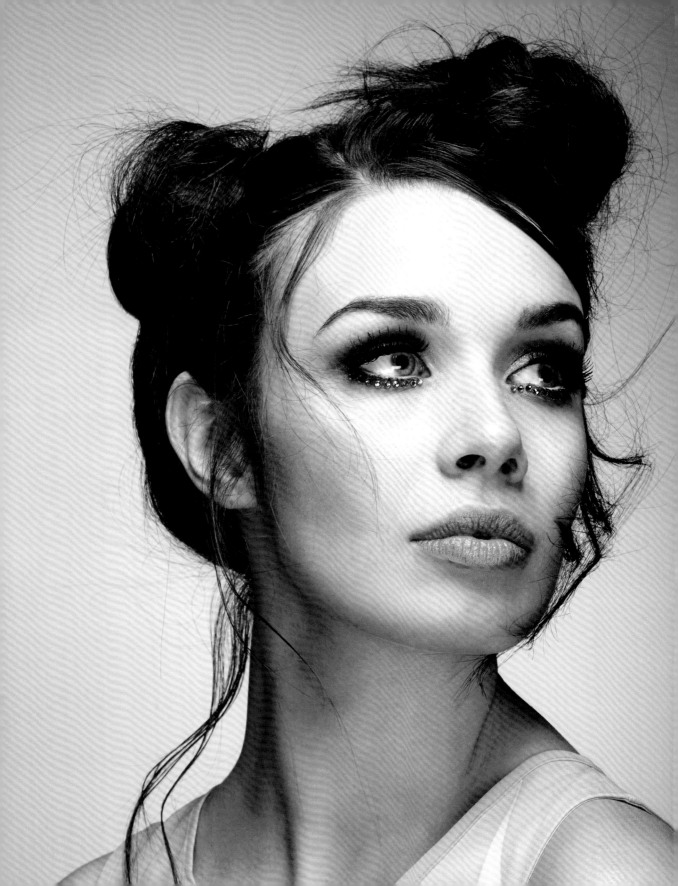

It's a bling thing in 30 minutes

Diamonds are a girl's best friend. Yes, they are indeed! So why not use them in a make-up look? Crystals look amazing over liner looks, or as an embellishment to a smoky eye.

For this look, I'm going to show you how to enhance a smoky eye with crystals by applying them like a liner under the lower lash line. Perfect your base and do a complete Classic smoky eye in 5, 15 or 30 minutes (see pages 48–51, 62–65 and 74–77). Then, ding, ding, it's time to bling!

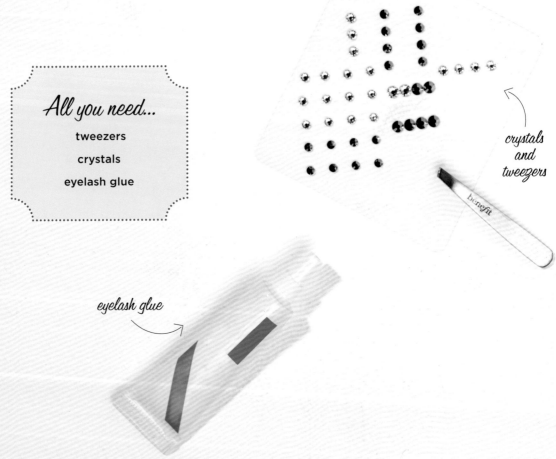

All you need...

tweezers

crystals

eyelash glue

crystals and tweezers

eyelash glue

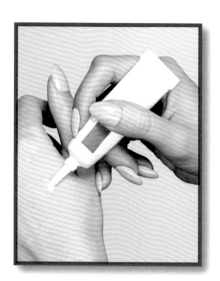

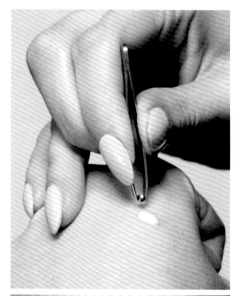

Going for gold

You can get small crystals from craft or bead shops and specialist companies like Swarovski.

Step 1

Apply a small amount of lash glue to the back of your hand to make it easier to dip the crystals in adhesive.

Step 2

Using tweezers, carefully pick up a crystal and dip the back of it into the lash glue. Allow it to dry for at least 30 seconds or until tacky.

Step 3

Look straight ahead into a mirror and, starting from the outer corner of your eye, carefully apply the crystals under the bottom lashes. Turn the tweezers over and use the flat edge to push the crystals in place. Hold for about 10 seconds, or until they are secure.

Keep applying the crystals in a row until you reach the end of the eye. Crystal eyes complete.

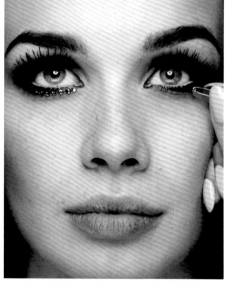

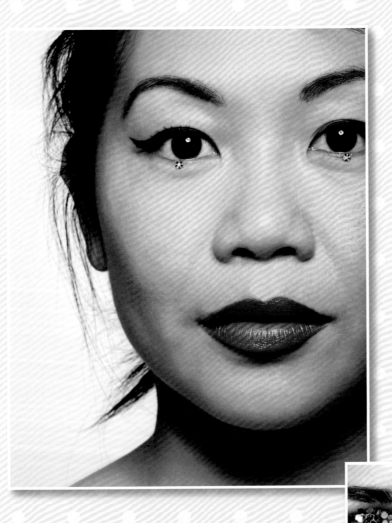

Alternative crystal eyes...

One crystal under the lower lash line looks super-cool. Perfect for a festival or night out.

Okay, these aren't crystals they're sequins. You can buy them in any fabric shop or online. Stick them on with Vaseline jelly, or, for a long-lasting finish, use a small amount of lash glue. I'm transporting you back to my disco-dancing days!

Resources

beautyblender®
www.beautyblender.com

Benefit Cosmetics
www.benefitcosmetics.co.uk

Boots
www.boots.com

Crown Brush
www.crownbrush.co.uk

DUO®
www.duoadhesives.com

Lisa Potter-Dixon for Benefit
www.lisapotterdixon.com

Lucas' Papaw Remedies
www.lucaspapaw.com.au

Make Up For Ever
www.makeupforever.com

OPI Products Inc.
www.opi.com

Sephora
www.sephora.com

Tweezerman®
www.tweezerman.com

Vita Coco®
www.vitacoco.com

Essential tools

beautyblender® Classic
Benefit foundation brush
Benefit blush brush
Benefit hard-angle brush
Make Up For Ever Precision
   Blender Brush – Medium 216
Crown Brush Infinity Blending
   Fluff C460
Crown Brush Pro Blending
   Crease C441
DUO® Striplash Adhesive
   White/Clear
Tweezerman® Slant Tweezer
Nails OPI *Chillin' Like a Villain*.

All you need... (in detail)

14 Benefit: the POREfessional; hello flawless! oxygen wow *believe in me (ivory)*; gimme brow *medium/deep*; they're real! mascara *black*; dandelion; hydra-smooth lip colour *air kiss.*

16–17 Benefit: foamingly clean facial wash; instant comeback serum; total moisture facial cream; it's potent! eye cream. Vita Coco®: Coconut Oil

18 Benefit: the POREfessional; that gal; girl meets pearl.

19 Benefit: stay don't stray *light/medium.*

20–21 Benefit: hello flawless! oxygen wow *I'm so money (honey)*; the POREfessional: agent zero shine.

22 Benefit: it's potent! eye cream; boi-ing *02.*

23 Benefit: hello flawless! oxygen wow *I'm so money (honey)*; fakeup *01.*

24 Benefit: that gal; hello flawless! oxygen wow *I'm so money (honey)*; stay don't stray *light/medium*; fakeup *01*; hoola; hervana; roller lash mascara; brow zings *dark*; gimme brow *medium/deep*; hydra-smooth lip colour *air kiss.* Make Up For Ever: Diamond Powder *2 White Gold.*

25 (clockwise from top left) Benefit: CORALista; sugarbomb; hervana.

30–31 Benefit: the POREfessional; hello flawless! oxygen wow *I'm pure for sure (ivory)*; fakeup *01*; hoola; posietint, sun beam; they're real! mascara *black*; gimme brow *medium/deep*; speed brow; posiebalm.

32 Benefit: the POREfessional; hello flawless! oxygen wow *I'm pure for sure (ivory)*; stay don't stray *light/medium*; sugarbomb; roller lash mascara; brow zings *dark*; gimme brow *medium/deep.*

33 (top left) Benefit: the POREfessional; hello flawless! oxygen wow *cheers to me (champagne)*; fakeup *01*; hoola; sugarbomb; big beautiful eyes; they're real push-up liner *black*; roller lash mascara; gimme brow *medium/deep*; benebalm.

33 (bottom right) Benefit: the POREfessional; boi-ing *05*; they're real push-up liner *blue*; they're real mascara *blue*; instant brow pencil *deep*; gimme brow *medium/deep*; benetint. Make Up For Ever: HD Foundation *178 Chestnut*; HD Blush *520 Blackcurrant.* Vaseline jelly.

36–37 Benefit: they're real! mascara *black*

38–40 Benefit: girl meets pearl; hello flawless! oxygen wow *I'm so money (honey)*; erase paste *1*; hoola; hervana; they're real! mascara *black*; BADgal liner waterproof *black*; brow zings *dark*; gimme brow *medium/deep*; pinup lash.

41 Benefit: girl meets pearl; hello flawless! oxygen wow *all the world's my stage (beige)*; hoola; hervana; they're real! mascara *black*; gimme brow *medium/deep*; cha cha balm; starlet lash.

42–43 Benefit: the POREfessional; hello flawless! oxygen wow *I'm so money (honey)*; longwear powder shadow *kiss me, I'm tipsy*; roller lash mascara; going solo lash.

44–45 Benefit: girl meets pearl; hello flawless! oxygen wow *I'm so money (honey)*; hoola; they're real! push-up liner *black*; they're real! mascara *black.*

46 Benefit: girl meets pearl; BADgal liner waterproof *black*; they're real! mascara *black.* Dior: Diorskin Star *dark brown.* Make Up For Ever: HD Blush *510 Raspberry*; Artist Shadow – Iridescent Finish *I-220 Sapphire*; Artist Shadow – Diamond Finish *D-222 Night Blue.* Lucas' Papaw Ointment.

48–51 Benefit: that gal; hello flawless! oxygen wow *believe in me (ivory)*; fakeup *01*; posietint; brow zings *dark*;

they're real! mascara *black*. **Make Up For Ever**: Artist Shadow – Matte Finish *M-110 Cement*.

52-54 Benefit: the POREfessional; hello flawless! oxygen wow *what I crave (toasted beige)*; boi-ing *03*; hoola; posietint; they're real! push-up liner *black*; they're real! mascara *black*; gimme brow *medium/deep*; hoola ultra plush. **Make Up For Ever**: Artist Shadow – Diamond Finish *D-652 Celestrial Earth*.

55 Benefit: the POREfessional; hello flawless! oxygen wow *cheers to me (champagne)*; fakeup *01*; hoola; CORALista; they're real! mascara *black*; benetint; gimme brow *medium/deep*. **Make Up For Ever**: Artist Shadow – Diamond Finish *D-652 Celestrial Earth*.

56-59 Benefit: the POREfessional; hello flawless! oxygen wow *believe in me (ivory)*; dandelion; creaseless cream shadow *always a bridesmaid*; they're real! mascara *blue*; brow zings *dark*; speed brow. **Make Up For Ever**: Rouge Artist Natural *N31 Soft Fuchsia*.

60-61 Benefit: hello flawless! oxygen wow *I'm so money (honey)*; hoola; hydra-smooth lip colour *lip service*; they're real! push-up liner *blue*; they're real! mascara *blue*; ultra plush lip gloss *icebreaker*.

62-65 Benefit: hello flawless! oxygen wow *I'm pure for sure (ivory)*; hoola; hervana; sun beam; smokin' eyes; they're real! mascara *black*; BADgal liner waterproof *black*.

66-68 Benefit: girl meets pearl; hello flawless! oxygen wow *I'm so money (honey)*; erase paste *1*; hoola; CORALista; longwear powder shadow *gilt-y pleasure* and *kiss me, I'm tipsy*; BADgal liner waterproof *espresso*; they're real! mascara *black*; gimme brow *medium/deep*; ultra plush lip gloss *fauxmance*. **Make Up For Ever**: Artist Shadow – Diamond Finish *D-708 Pinky Copper*.

69 Benefit: the POREfessional; hello

flawless! oxygen wow *I'm pure for sure (ivory)*; fakeup *01*; hoola; dallas; longwear powder shadow *kiss me, I'm tipsy*; BADgal liner waterproof *black*; they're real! mascara *black*; brow zings *dark*; gimme brow *medium/deep*; boi-ing *01*. **Make Up For Ever**: Artist Shadow – Diamond Finish *D-652 Celestrial Earth*.

70-73 Benefit: that gal; hello flawless! oxygen wow *believe in me (ivory)*; High Beam; dandelion; roller lash mascara; gimme brow *medium/deep*; posietint; boi-ing *02*. **Make Up For Ever**: Artist Shadow – Diamond Finish *D-236 Lagoon Blue*; Artist Shadow – Iridescent Finish *I-300 Pine Green*.

74-77 Benefit: girl meets pearl; hello flawless! oxygen wow *I'm pure for sure (ivory)*; hoola; hervana; boi-ing *01*; stay don't stray *light/medium*; smokin' eyes; eye bright pencil; they're real! mascara *black*; they're real! push-up liner *black*; brow zings *dark*; gimme brow *medium/deep*; benetint. **Make Up For Ever**: Artist Shadow – Matte Finish *M-100 Black*; Star Powder *940 White with orange highlights*.

78-81 Benefit: girl meets pearl; hello flawless! oxygen wow *I'm so money (honey)*; boi-ing *02*; hoola; dallas; longwear powder shadow *gilt-y pleasure* and *kiss me, I'm tipsy*; they're real! push-up liner *black*; they're real! mascara *black*; pinup lash; speed brow; hydra-smooth lip colour *air kiss*. **Make Up For Ever**: Artist Shadow – Metallic Finish *ME-728 Copper Red*; Artist Shadow – Diamond Finish *D-320 Golden Khaki*.

82 Benefit: girl meets pearl; hello flawless! oxygen wow *believe in me (ivory)*; boi-ing *02*; hoola; hervana; longwear powder shadow *gilt-y pleasure* and *kiss me, I'm tipsy*; they're real! push-up liner *black*; they're real! mascara *black*; pinup lash; gimme brow *medium/deep*; ultra plush lip gloss *icebreaker*. **Make Up For Ever**: Artist Shadow – Metallic Finish *ME-*

728 Copper Red; Artist Shadow – Diamond Finish *D-320 Golden Khaki*.

83 Benefit: the POREfessional; hello flawless! oxygen wow *I'm pure for sure (ivory)*; fakeup *01*; sugarbomb; longwear powder shadow *gilt-y pleasure* and *kiss me, I'm tipsy*; they're real! push-up liner *black*; they're real! mascara *black*; pinup lash; speed brow; cha cha tint; ultra plush lip gloss *icebreaker*. **Make Up For Ever**: Artist Shadow – Metallic Finish *ME-728 Copper Red*; Shadow – Diamond Finish *D-320 Golden Khaki*.

84-87 Benefit: hello flawless! oxygen wow *I'm pure for sure (ivory)*; erase paste *1*; hoola; bella bamba; sun beam; they're real! mascara *black*; they're real! push-up liner *black*; BADgal liner waterproof *black*; pinup lash; gimme brow *medium/deep*. **Make Up For Ever**: Artist Shadow – Iridescent Finish *I-858 Flamingo*, *I-922 Electric Purple* and *I-220 Sapphire*. **Lucas' Papaw Ointment**.

88 Benefit: that gal; hello flawless! oxygen wow I'm so money (honey); hoola; CORALista; they're real! push-up liner black; brow zings dark. **Lucas' Papaw Ointment**.

90-92 Benefit: girl meets pearl; hello flawless! oxygen wow *I'm so money (honey)*; fakeup *01*; hoola; hervana; they're real! push-up liner *black*; roller lash mascara; gimme brow *medium/deep*; ultra plush lip gloss *poutrageous!*.

93 Benefit: that gal; hello flawless! oxygen wow *I'm so money (honey)*; hoola; CORALista; they're real! push-up liner *black*; brow zings dark; cha cha balm.

94-96 Benefit: hello flawless! oxygen wow *I'm pure for sure (ivory)*; stay don't stray *light/medium*; hoola; posietint; High Beam; they're real! push-up liner *black*; they're real! mascara *black* and *blue*; brow zings *dark*; cha cha tint; cha cha balm. **Make Up For Ever**: Artist Shadow

– Satiny Finish *S-312 Mint Green*.

97 Benefit: the POREfessional; hello flawless! oxygen wow *I'm so money (honey)*; boi-ng *02*; hoola; hervana; they're real! push-up liner *purple*; they're real! mascara *black*.

98–100 Benefit: girl meets pearl; hello flawless! oxygen wow *warm me up (toasted beige)*; boi-ing *03*; hoola; majorette; BADgal liner waterproof *black*; roller lash mascara; brow zings *dark*; hoola ultra plush.

101 Benefit: the POREfessional; hello flawless! oxygen wow *cheers to me (champagne)*; fakeup *01*; hoola; CORALista; eye bright pencil; roller lash mascara; posietint; gimme brow *medium/deep*.

104–107 Benefit: that gal; hello flawless! oxygen wow *I'm so money (honey)*; fakeup *01*; hoola; CORALista; they're real! push-up liner *black*; brow zings *dark*; cha cha balm.

108 Benefit: girl meets pearl; hello flawless! oxygen wow *I'm all the rage (beige)*; fakeup *02*; hoola; hervana; they're real! push-up liner *green*; roller lash mascara; gimme brow *medium/deep*.

109 Benefit: the POREfessional; hello flawless! oxygen wow *I'm so money (honey)*; fakeup *02*; hoola; majorette; stay don't stray *light/medium*; they're real! push-up liner *black*; they're real! mascara *black*; high brow; gimme brow *medium/deep*; CORALista ultra plush.

110–112 Benefit: that gal; hello flawless! oxygen wow *I'm pure for sure (ivory)*; fakeup *01*; dandelion; gimme brow *medium/deep*; majorette. **Make Up For Ever:** Artist Shadow – Iridescent Finish *I-858 Flamingo*. Vaseline jelly.

113 Benefit: the POREfessional; hello flawless! oxygen wow *believe in me (ivory)*; fakeup *01*; High Beam; they're real! push-up liner *black*; they're real! mascara *black*; brow zings *dark*; gimme brow *medium/deep*; cha cha tint; cha cha balm.

114–116 Benefit: girl meets pearl; hello flawless! oxygen wow *I'm all the rage (beige)*; fakeup *02*; CORALista; they're real! push-up liner *blue*; roller lash; gimme brow *medium/deep*. **Make Up For Ever:** Aqua Lip *16C Fuchsia*; Artist Plexi-gloss *209 Fuchsia Pink*.

117 Benefit: girl meets pearl; hello flawless! oxygen wow *warm me up (toasted beige)*; boi-ing *03*; hoola; hervana; they're real! push-up liner *blue*; brow zings *dark*; hoola. **Make Up For Ever:** Artist Shadow – Diamond Finish *D-222 Night Blue*.

118–120 Benefit: girl meets pearl; hello flawless! oxygen wow *I'm pure for sure (ivory)*; boi-ing *01*; hoola; hervana; stay don't stray *light/medium*; they're real! push-up liner *black*; BADgal liner waterproof *black*; they're real! mascara *black*; gimme brow *medium/deep*; posiebalm.

122 Benefit: girl meets pearl; hello flawless! oxygen wow *I'm pure for sure (ivory)*; hoola; hervana; bo-ing *01*; stay don't stray *light/medium*; smokin' eyes; they're real! mascara *black*; eye bright pencil; BADgal liner waterproof *black*; pinup lash; Bling Brow; brow zings *dark*; gimme brow *medium/deep*; cha cha tint; boi-ing *01*.

124–127 Benefit: the POREfessional; hello flawless! oxygen wow *I'm pure for sure (ivory)*; boi-ing *01*; sugarbomb; longwear powder shadow *kiss me, I'm tipsy*; BADgal liner waterproof *black*; they're real! mascara *black*; gimme brow *light/medium*; ultra plush lip gloss *icebreaker*. Vaseline jelly. **Make Up For Ever:** Diamond Powder *15 Smoky*.

128 Benefit: the POREfessional; hello flawless! oxygen wow *I'm so money (honey)*; hoola; dandelion; stay don't stray *light/medium*; roller lash mascara; brow zings *dark*; gimme brow *medium/ deep*; hoola ultra plush. **Make Up For Ever:** Diamond Powder *2 White Gold*.

129 Benefit: girl meets pearl; hello flawless! oxygen wow *warm me up (toasted beige)*; boi-ing *03*; hoola; hervana; longwear powder shadow *raincheck?*; they're real! push-up liner *blue*; they're real! mascara *black*; gimme brow *medium/deep*; ultra plush lip gloss *lollibop*. **Make Up For Ever:** Diamond Powder *14 Baby Mauve*.

130–131 Benefit: hello flawless! oxygen wow *I'm pure for sure (ivory)*; the POREfessional: agent zero shine; hoola; ultra plush lip gloss *icebreaker*; they're real! mascara *black*; gimme brow *medium/deep*. **Make Up For Ever:** Rouge Artist Intense *22 Satin Nude*.

132 Benefit: girl meets pearl; hello flawless! oxygen wow *I'm so money (honey)*; boi-ing *02*; hoola; posietint; smokin' eyes; they're real! mascara *black*; ultra plush lip gloss *icebreaker*; gimme brow *medium/deep*; posietint.

136–138 Benefit: girl meets pearl; hello flawless! oxygen wow *I'm pure for sure (ivory)*; hoola; hervana; bo-ing *01*; stay don't stray *light/medium*; smokin' eyes; they're real! mascara *black*; eye bright pencil; BADgal liner waterproof *black*; pinup lash; Bling Brow; brow zings *dark*; gimme brow *medium/deep*; cha cha tint; boi-ing *01*.

139 (top) Benefit: girl meets pearl; hello flawless! oxygen wow *I'm all the rage (beige)*; fakeup *02*; CORALista; they're real! push-up liner *blue*; roller lash mascara; Bling Brow; gimme brow *medium/deep*. **Make Up For Ever:** Aqua Lip *16C Fuchsia*; Artist Plexi-gloss *209 Fuchsia Pink*.

139 (bottom) Benefit: girl meets pearl; hello flawless! oxygen wow *I'm pure for sure (ivory)*; hoola; hervana; bo-ing *01*; stay don't stray *light/medium*; they're real! mascara *black*; pinup lash; gimme brow *medium/deep*; cha cha balm; ultra plush lip gloss *icebreaker*. Vaseline jelly. **Make Up For Ever:** Extra Large Size Glitters *N01 Gold*.

Index

Acknowledgments

I've loved every second of creating this book. It's been an incredible journey, but I couldn't have done it without the love and support of a lot of people...

To my Theo. For hot baths, coffees, Kinder eggs and everything else in between. You inspire me every day. I love you, x.

Snoopy and Kimmy, you're the best! Even if you did walk, sleep and wee on this book as I was trying to write it!

To my Benefit Family, you guys drive me to be the best that I can be. Your constant support is invaluable. Gail, Ian and Andrea, thank you for always believing in me and my crazy ideas. Hannah, we made it! This wouldn't have happened without your support and advice. Thank you!

Lauren, the greatest make-up assistant, break dancer and triangle face-maker in the game. I couldn't do my job without you. You're the best!

To everyone at Ryland Peters & Small, thanks for seeking me out, and thank you for all your continued support in making this epic project happen! BIG thank you to Julia, Leslie, Steph, Sonya and Luis for being there every step of the way.

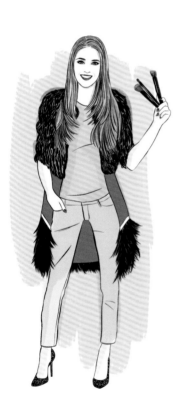

To the #EasyOnTheEyes dream team: Tom Andrew (snaps), David Wadlow (hurrr) and John Philip Heyes (lighting and tea), you guys have made this one of the best experiences of my life. From the Hackney bake off to the Pajama party of dreams, thanks for seeing my vision and blowing it up.

To the beautiful ladies in my life: Mum, Mumpen, Nan, Nanna Potter, Patricia, Dawny, Deb, Dani, Janice, Jenna, Lucy, Kate, Emi, Esme, Georgie, Hannah, Rosie, Emzie, Caz, Clare, Tana, Franny, Faye, Alexa, Dawny, Kirsi, Ashley, Laura, Sophie, Carrie, Annaliese, Alex, Clare Gater, Kate, Kyra, Laurretta, Tanny, Neens, Winny, JP, JS, Lorna, Michelle, Claire, Amy-Lou, Alyson, Jazz, Bridget, Sophie B, Liv, Julia, Becci, Megan, Helen, Tux, Carina, Amy, Nicky and baby Esmae.

To the men: Dad, Grandad, Norman, Eric, Peter, Ian, Bob, Jack, Steve, Eddie, Joe, Ben, Riley, Blake, Elliot, Ed, Julio, Jordan, Hamish, Mungo, Liam, Sam, Nick, Bry, Simsy, Dan, Blackers, Ollie, Ludo, Mike, Neil, George, Ed, Kev, Kas, Dano, Carlos, Mark, JM, Jay, Ben, Leon, Dom, Andy and Jamie.

You are all incredible. I am who I am because of you lot. My life would be boring without the fun, laughter and craziness you bring.

Sally Cotterill, your talent as an illustrator blows me away. Thank you for all your colourful creativity. You have made my book extra-beautiful. @sally_faye.

All hail my nails! To the man who's changing the nail game, Michael Do. Thanks for keeping my nails looking incredible for the book. @Michaeldo92.

Tom and Ashley, aka 'TPAK'. Two of the hardest-working people I know. Thank you for the LFW pics and for the behind-the-scenes video. Legends!

Lorraine, Matthew, Jo, thank you for your wonderfully kind words for this book. I'll be forever grateful for the chances you have taken on me.

To all the hard-working make-up artists out there! You all inspire me every day.

To the models and real women that you see on these pages, and to all the women I have ever worked with. Thank you for letting me paint your beautiful faces.